Praise for *The*

"I am amazed at how easy *The S[...]*
incredibly nutritious food to your d[...]
entrepreneur, *New York Times* bestselling author of
***Living with a SEAL*, and co-owner of the Atlanta Hawks**

"Sprouts are an incredible and versatile food that anyone can grow at home. This book provides the background, inspiration, and instruction for making sprouts part of your daily life. I highly recommend it!"
—Katie Wells, founder of WellnessMama.com

"Doug Evans shows how easy and wildly affordable it is to eat the healthiest foods on the planet. Anyone looking to energize their body and upgrade their health needs this book." **—Vani Hari, *New York Times* bestselling author and founder of FoodBabe.com**

"Doug Evans reveals the mysterious genius of plant intelligence. . . . In *The Sprout Book*, he demonstrates and guides us to understand . . . the raw nutritious miracles that exist in the cycle of life."
—Deepak Chopra, *New York Times* bestselling author of
Metahuman: Unleashing Your Infinite Potential

"Sprouting foods can add to their nutritional value. In this comprehensive yet easily accessible book, Doug Evans shows you how and why." **—Dean Ornish, M.D., author of *Undo It***

"Sprouts can be a fun and affordable way to access fresh food. *The Sprout Book* will show you how to bring sprouts to life in your own home." **—Brian Wendel, president of Forks Over Knives**

"Is there a nutritious, easy to produce, easy to grow, absolutely effective food category that we can all agree is wonderful? Let's all get together with Doug Evans and eat more sprouts!" **—David Avocado Wolfe, author of *The Sunfood Diet Success System*, *Eating for Beauty*, and *Chaga: King of the Medicinal Mushrooms***

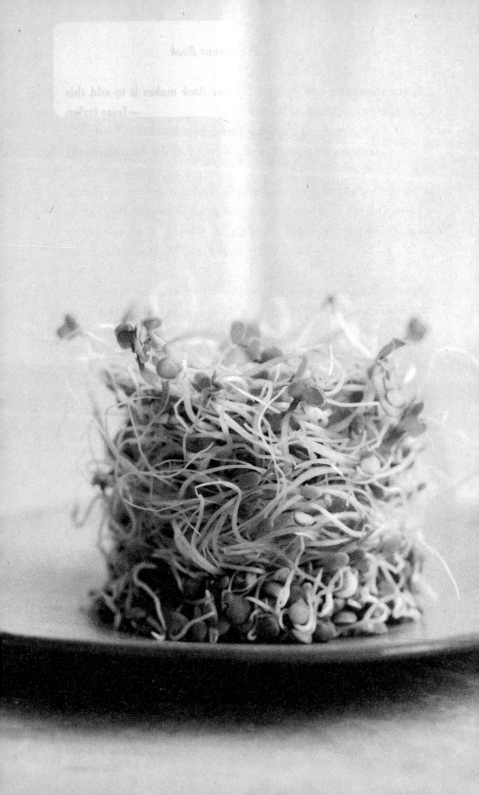

THE
SPROUT
BOOK

Tap into the Power of
the Planet's Most Nutritious Food

DOUG EVANS

with Leda Scheintaub
Foreword by Joel Fuhrman, M.D.

ST. MARTIN'S
ESSENTIALS
NEW YORK

First published in the United States by St. Martin's Essentials,
an imprint of St. Martin's Publishing Group

THE SPROUT BOOK. Copyright © 2020 by Doug Evans. Foreword copyright © 2020 by Joel Fuhrman. All rights reserved. Printed in the United States of America. For information, address St. Martin's Publishing Group, 120 Broadway, New York, NY 10271.

www.stmartins.com

Photograph courtesy of Clare Barboza Photography

Designed by Steven Seighman

Library of Congress Cataloging-in-Publication Data

Names: Evans, Doug, author.
Title: The sprout book: tap into the power of the planet's most nutritious
   food / Doug Evans.
Description: First edition. | New York: St. Martin's Essentials, 2020. |
   Includes bibliographical references and index.
Identifiers: LCCN 2019047192 | ISBN 9781250226174 (trade paperback) |
   ISBN 9781250226181 (ebook)
Subjects: LCSH: Sprouts. | Cooking (Sprouts)
Classification: LCC SB324.53 .E93 2020 | DDC 641.6/536—dc23
LC record available at https://lccn.loc.gov/2019047192

Our books may be purchased in bulk for promotional, educational, or business use. Please contact your local bookseller or the Macmillan Corporate and Premium Sales Department at 1-800-221-7945, extension 5442, or by email at MacmillanSpecialMarkets@macmillan.com.

First Edition: April 2020

11 13 15 17 19 20 18 16 14 12

This book is dedicated to all of the plant- and animal-loving people who care about the Earth and each other.
To my late mother and father, Beverly and Robert, who had so much love for me and made so many sacrifices so that I could lead the life that I live.
To my brother, Andrew, who is my greatest teacher and is always there for me.
To my beloved Sivan, who inspires me every day to be the best version of myself.

CONTENTS

FOREWORD

We are in an era of scientific advancements enabling prolongation of human life via nutritional excellence.

In other words, it has not been advancements in medicine, pharmacology, surgical techniques, radiation, and organ transplantation that have offered our population a dramatic difference in extending healthy life expectancy; rather it has been diet and nutrition that enable dramatic potential for a healthful and lengthy life, in spite of it generally being ignored by health professionals and the public. It is living in a manner that enables us to be so healthy that we can avoid health care that leads to excellent health, not access to health care.

I always say, "We have landed a man on the moon already!" And by that, I mean we already know how to save millions of lives, win the war on cancer, and protect our population from heart attacks and strokes—the leading causes of death. The answer is *vegetables*. People don't like that answer. They are still seeking a magic pill they can take so they can still smoke cigarettes and not get lung cancer or think they can eat pizza, hot dogs, doughnuts, and bagels and not get breast cancer. Life is not a fairy tale. In the real world, we are formed from what we ate in our lives, and we have the full rights and responsibility to destroy our health with unhealthy foods or protect it with nutritious, healthy plant foods.

Given the depth of scientific studies on this issue, and the power of nutrition to unleash the miraculous healing powers in our cells, it is evident that we have an unprecedented opportunity in human history to live longer and better than ever before, if, and only if, we choose to eat an ideal diet.

I am an outspoken advocate of a Nutritarian diet—a nutrient-dense, plant-rich diet that includes a wide variety of natural plant foods with their rich phytonutrient, anti-inflammatory, and anticancer benefits. A Nutritarian diet also recommends greens, beans, mushrooms, onions, berries, and seeds for their varying and synergistic anticancer and life span benefits.

Clean green foods are the secret to a long, healthy life. Greens not only fuel our cells' major repair mechanisms, they are also needed for the normal functioning of our immune systems. Greens suppress genetic alterations that, if left exposed, could contribute to cancer development.

For example, green cruciferous plants enable the production of isothiocyanates (ITCs), formed when the cell wall is broken as the food is eaten or blended. The cruciferous family is unique among vegetables because of their glucosinolate content; glucosinolates give cruciferous vegetables their characteristic spicy or bitter tastes. When the plant cell walls are broken by blending, chopping, or chewing, an enzyme called *my-*

rosinase converts glucosinolates to isothiocyanates (ITCs)—compounds with potent anticancer effects, including:*

- Anti-inflammatory effects—ITCs have been found to decrease the secretion of inflammatory molecules.
- Anti-angiogenic effects—Isothiocyanates can inhibit the development of new blood vessels to limit tumor growth.
- Detoxification of carcinogens—Some carcinogens must be converted to their active form before they can bind to DNA to cause carcinogenic changes; isothiocyanates can block this transformation.
- Preventing DNA damage—Isothiocyanates also increase the production of the body's natural detoxification enzymes, which protect DNA against damage from carcinogens and free radicals.
- Stopping cell division in cells whose DNA has been damaged.
- Promoting programmed cell death in cancerous cells.
- Anti-estrogenic activity—Exposure to estrogen is known to increase breast cancer risk; estrogens can alter gene expression, promoting cell proliferation in breast tissue. ITCs have been shown to inhibit the expression of estrogen-responsive genes.
- Shifting hormone metabolism—Eating cruciferous vege-

---

* J. Higdon, B. Delage, D. Williams, et al., "Cruciferous Vegetables and Human Cancer Risk: Epidemiologic Evidence and Mechanistic Basis," *Pharmacological Research* 55, no. 3 (2007): 224–236.

tables regularly helps the body to shift hormone metabolism, reducing the cancer-promoting potency of estrogen and other hormones.

Eating cruciferous vegetables produces measurable isothiocyanates in breast tissue,[*] and observational studies show that women who eat more cruciferous vegetables are less likely to be diagnosed with breast cancer. In a recent Chinese study, women who regularly ate one serving per day of cruciferous vegetables had a 50 percent reduced risk of breast cancer.[†] A 17 percent decrease in breast cancer risk was found in a European study for consuming cruciferous vegetables at least once a week.[‡]

The new study kept track of cruciferous vegetable intake in Chinese women with breast cancer for the first three years after diagnosis, and followed the women for a total of five years. They found dose-response effects—this means that the more cruciferous vegetables women ate, the less likely they were to experience breast cancer recurrence or die from breast cancer. When the women were grouped into four quartiles of cruciferous vegetable consumption, those in the highest quartile had a

---

[*] B. S. Cornblatt, L. Ye, A. T. Dinkova-Kostova, et al., "Preclinical and Clinical Evaluation of Sulforaphane for Chemoprevention in the Breast," *Carcinogenesis* 28, no. 7 (2007): 1485–1490.

[†] C. X. Zhang, S. C. Ho, Y. M. Chen, et al., "Greater Vegetable and Fruit Intake Is Associated with a Lower Risk of Breast Cancer Among Chinese Women," *International Journal of Cancer* 125, no. 1 (2009): 181–188.

[‡] C. Bosetti, M. Filomeno, P. Riso, et al., "Cruciferous Vegetables and Cancer Risk in a Network of Case-Control Studies," *Annals of Oncology* 23, no. 8 (2012): 2198–2203.

62 percent decrease in risk of death and 35 percent reduced risk of recurrence compared to the lowest quartile.[*]

This new data supports a previous report from the Women's Healthy Eating and Living (WHEL) Study. Breast cancer survivors who reported higher than median cruciferous vegetable intake and were in the top third of total vegetable intake had a 52 percent reduced risk of recurrence—especially powerful since the average intakes were quite low—3.1 and 0.5 servings/day of total and cruciferous vegetables, respectively.[†]

The message and point here is that food is powerful, and greens are likely the most powerful food you can eat to prevent cancer and prolong life span. This healing power is even more concentrated in young vegetables, sprouts, and microgreens. These tiny powerhouses are secret weapons in the war on cancer, as they enable us to optimize our ITC exposure so easily and without high cost or risk of pesticides or contamination. Sprouts and microgreens are inexpensive, can be made at home, and can add the benefits of green superfoods to almost everyone's diet.

Despite being low in calories, sprouts are a rich source of nutrients and beneficial plant compounds. Their vitamin and mineral content is high. The sprouting process increases nutrient levels,

---

[*] S. J. Nechuta, W. Lu, H. Cai, et al., "Cruciferous Vegetable Intake After Diagnosis of Breast Cancer and Survival: A Report from the Shanghai Breast Cancer Survival Study. Abstract #LB-322," Annual Meeting of the American Association for Cancer Research, March 31–April 4, 2012, Chicago, Illinois.

[†] C. A. Thomson, C. L. Rock, P. A. Thompson, et al., "Vegetable Intake Is Associated with Reduced Breast Cancer Recurrence in Tamoxifen Users: A Secondary Analysis from the Women's Healthy Eating and Living Study," *Breast Cancer Research and Treatment* 125, no. 2 (2011): 519–527.

making sprouts richer in protein, folate, magnesium, phosphorus, manganese, and vitamins C and K than un-sprouted plants.

That means that sprouts have higher levels of amino acids that may be low in starchy vegetables and grains, with specific amino acids increasing by as much as 30 percent. And the proteins in sprouts are also easier to digest than the proteins in beans and nuts and seeds. The sprouting process also reduces the amount of antinutrients, such as phytic acid, that decrease your body's ability to absorb nutrients from the plant—by up to 87 percent. So the minerals in sprouts are more absorbable. Sprouts are also great sources of antioxidants and other beneficial plant compounds.

We have a choice today. We can eat super healthfully with the best scientifically supported and protective foods to enable great health and protect ourselves from having a tragic future, or we can eat the worst diet ever available and have heart disease and strokes and get cancer. It's up to you. I'm certainly rooting for you and hoping you read this book, sprout and grow greens, and get and stay healthy.

Joel Fuhrman, M.D.
Six-time New York Times *bestselling author*
DrFuhrman.com

INTRODUCTION: BACK TO THE SEED

FOR THE LAST twenty years, I have been searching for the perfect food. I started as a fast-food- and meat-eater raised on the Standard American Diet on the streets of New York City. I understood early on that vegetables were good for you, yet I ate candy, pizza, pasta, hamburgers, milkshakes, cheese, ribs, and, of course, fried chicken. The less healthy the food was, the more I was attracted to it. After three different high schools, spray-painting graffiti on hundreds of subway trains, and causing all kinds of ruckus, I joined the U.S. Army's Eighty-Second Airborne Division as the lowest-ranking enlisted soldier to jump out of planes and run through the woods. The army was a turning point in my life, because it taught me discipline and built my confidence, two traits that would serve me well in taking control of my life and my health. After the army, I turned my passion for street art into one of the first digital printing and graphic design studios. I developed an obsession for technology and went on to work with Paul Rand and Apple, Microsoft, and Adobe Systems.

Then my life changed forever when I watched my mother die of cancer at sixty-six and then my father die at age seventy-seven of heart disease in the same hospital. My mother's sister had died from cancer, and her husband died of heart disease. Her brother died of heart disease, and his wife died of complications from diabetes. And my older brother became morbidly obese, developed type 2 diabetes, heart disease, and atrial fibrillation, and had the first of three strokes.

At age twenty-nine, I really thought my life was doomed. That I was dealt a bad hand of genes and I should get my affairs in order. Thank goddess, a random (nothing is really random) event introduced me to my first vegan friend, Denise Mari, at 2:00 a.m. in a New York City nightclub. I literally went from eating anything to exclusively eating raw fruits and vegetables within the space of two weeks.

I began to see the world in a completely different way. It was like when I was in second grade and I put on my glasses for the first time. Suddenly, everything was clear. Until I took one of those eye chart tests, I thought that I could see like everybody else. As I watched the other kids see all the smallest letters and numbers, I could see that even with my best squinting, I was outmatched. As I sat in the optometrist's chair and watched the various lenses being flipped, the chart kept getting clearer and clearer. Occasionally, it would get worse and I would squelch, and then I would get closer to divine perfection. The world was getting clear to me. Still, I hated my glasses. I feared being called *four eyes*. While walking down a single New York City block, I put my glasses on and took them off at least a dozen times, and after that, I didn't wear my glasses outside of the house for several years.

The relevance of that little story is that I knew that the glasses were good for me, but I let my aversion to them interfere with seeing perfectly, getting good grades, and even playing sports well. At Little League baseball, a ball literally hit me in the face because I couldn't see it coming.

That's the way it was for me with food, until my "cold cucumber" transformation. This was back in 1999 when the concept was almost unheard of. I quickly fell in love with nature. My entire world opened up. Losing weight literally and figuratively made me feel light and high on life. My chronic stuffy and bloody noses were gone, my crusty eyes were clear, and I could breathe clearly through both nostrils at the same time. My lower back pain was gone for good. It felt like a miracle. The challenge was what to eat, in what quantity, and where I was going to get it. Those were legitimate concerns, but I was focused, resourceful, and determined.

Every day, it became a little easier. I became familiar with how to adapt a menu in my local restaurants to accommodate me. I found foods that tasted good, filled me up, and digested well. Along the way, I experimented with some extreme forms of the diet. I ate mono fruitarian for a while. This meant eating exclusively fruit, one type at a time, until I was no longer hungry and then waiting a few hours until I was hungry and finding another fruit. It was fun, satisfying, and very effective. I loved it, and if I had lived in Bali or Hawaii, it would have been easy, but in my heart, I didn't feel it was necessary. Adding salads, vegetables, seaweeds, seeds, and nuts made it so much easier, and that became my inspiration behind the launch of my first plant-based business.

Armed with the knowledge that 90 percent of Americans weren't getting enough vegetables, in 2002, I invested in and cofounded (with Denise Mari) Organic Avenue, the first major organic cold-pressed juice and raw food retailer in the United States. We started the company in my loft in Chinatown, opened twelve stores across Manhattan, and grew more than 100 percent a year for ten years, until the sale of the company in 2012 to a private equity group. The goal of my next venture, Juicero, was to make a product that would enable people to load up on fresh, ripe, organic produce in an easily deliverable form. Five years, nine food scientists, twelve Ph.D.s, and fifty engineers later and the first at-home, cold-pressed juicing system was launched. By most measurements, Juicero was successful. We sold thousands of machines and more than a million Juicero packs, and the average Juicero user was consuming more than nine servings per week. But the company was sold to an investor group before hitting critical mass. After Juicero, I thought about what could serve the world better, and at a fraction of the cost. The answer was something I have been obsessively eating for the past two decades: sprouts! Everyone is looking for the fountain of youth. Some people spend up to a thousand dollars a day to stay at spas and retreat centers so they can get nourished with green drinks and plant-based cuisine, or they can do it at home, starting with sprouts. Sprouts are a nutrition revolution for everyone.

From Garnish to the Center of the Plate

In 1997, researchers at Johns Hopkins University discovered that broccoli sprouts contain astounding levels of cancer-protective chemicals. These chemicals, called *isothiocyanates,* make broccoli sprouts anywhere from thirty to fifty times more potent than mature broccoli. Since the discovery of the humble seed's potential, broccoli sprouts have reached superstardom in health-conscious circles, but most people in this country don't even know of their existence. Broccoli sprouts are still a niche of a niche, with far less than 1 percent of the U.S. population enjoying them on a regular basis.

Still, there is no shortage of great information about broccoli sprouts, but not so much for other sprouts. I believe that each living plant has something to teach us, and each sprout has its own story to tell. If as much money as went into researching broccoli sprouts went into a few other sprouts, I believe we would be amazed. But what we do know about sprouts is truly astounding, and without a doubt, there is no sustainable food on earth more nutritious than sprouts.

Sprouting brings new life to food, adding flavors and textures while packing in vitamins, micronutrients, phytonutrients, minerals, flavonoids, polyphenols, antioxidants, prebiotics, probiotics, and more. Sprouts are super low in calories (zero points on the Weight Watchers system!), low glycemic, and high in fiber and protein. Sprouting increases protein by as much as 20 percent and vitamins and other nutrients by up to 500 percent, making sprouts a healthier, unprocessed alternative to chalky, processed protein powders. Sprouting reduces phytic acid and lectins, substances found in beans and grains that can make them hard to digest. When beans and grains are sprouted, many people who gave them up are newly able to eat them. Sprouts are low in calories and high in everything that's good for us. We've all heard about Captain Cook's strategy of bringing citrus on board long sea voyages to keep his sailors from getting scurvy. What's even more interesting to me was learning that he also initiated a continuous program of growing and eating sprouts that was key to keeping the sailors well fed with vitamin C and avoiding death by scurvy.

For all intents and purposes, if you ate sprouts for breakfast, lunch, dinner, and a snack, you would barely get eight hundred calories into your system (and feel full) but the equivalent of three thousand to four thousand calories of nutrition relative to other foods. For example, my Super Green Sprout Smoothie (page 170) provides more nutrition from vitamins, minerals, and phytonutrients than many people get in a week! Sprouts fit in with popular diets, including Bulletproof, Keto, Atkins, Paleo, and more. Sprouting takes us back to the seed with an invitation to achieve our greatest health potential. *The Sprout Book* shares all that I've learned and gained from this superfood in one place.

You can safely make sprouts at home in two to seven days without specialized equipment. If you've heard scary stories about contaminated sprouts, not to worry. Sprouting is easy: You simply add water, then wait for nature's magical transformation from bean, grain, or seed to sprout. I will cover how much water to add, when to add, when to rinse, and when to refrigerate your sprouts to easily eliminate any chance of contamination.

Thanks to the increasing variety of sprouts available in natural food stores and supermarkets, it's easy to start a sprouting habit without going DIY. I'll share with you the best places to shop for sprouts, such as farmers' markets and natural food stores with a good turnover, and what to look for in terms of quality and freshness. In the span of my career, I've worked with produce production facilities from 400 to 111,000 square feet, and I am extremely experienced in properly handling fresh raw produce, including sprouts. I'll share from my experience how to shop for sprouts and provide my formula for cleaning sprouts so you can go forth and sprout safely and abundantly.

The goal of *The Sprout Book* is not only to nourish your body with this amazing plant food but to make magic in your kitchen. Sprouts add excitement to meals: adzuki, alfalfa, broccoli, buckwheat, cabbage, chia, chickpeas, clover, fenugreek, green pea, lentil, mung, mustard, onion, radish, sunflower . . . all these can be sprouted and offer up crisp, crunchy textures and tastes ranging from nutty to hardy, hot, crisp, powerful, sweet, and spicy. My goal with the recipes is to elevate sprouts from a garnish to the center of the plate and a catalyst for a radical shift in wellness.

Every recipe in the book is made up of a large percentage of sprouts. The rest will be raw vegetables, fruits, nuts, seeds, spices, sea vegetables, and top-quality oils. From takes on Indian street food to energizing green pea gazpacho, sophisticated lentil sprout pâté, and game-changing hummus, the recipes will blow your mind with flavor. All are simple to make, and none require a dehydrator, the stumbling block to many attempts at a raw food diet. You will learn that sprouts are a perfect food for training and that including sprout-based beverages can fuel your body with a plethora of macronutrients and micronutrients without the added sugar and artificial ingredients commonly found in sports drinks.

As you eat more sprouts as part of a plant-based diet, you will find yourself craving the pure burst of energy that a sprout smoothie, sprout salad, or a simple handful of sprouts delivers. You can expect to lose or maintain your weight while taking in more nutrition than ever, gaining energy, reducing inflammation, sleeping better, becoming more regular, and thinking more clearly. You can even tailor your sprout eating to supplement particular nutrients or target specific health conditions. This raw, living, plant-based way of eating is a deliciously low-cost, accessible way to heal the world, one seed at a time.

DR. DEAN ORNISH: "SPROUTS HAVE BENEFITS BEYOND THE NUTRIENTS THEY PROVIDE"

Dean Ornish, M.D., is the founder and president of the Preventive Medicine Research Institute and a leading expert on preventing and reversing heart disease with dietary and lifestyle changes including a whole-foods, plant-based diet. He has been a physician consultant to former president Bill Clinton and was appointed by former president Barack Obama to the Advisory Group on Prevention, Health Promotion, and Integrative and Public Health. He has written multiple bestsellers, including the classic *Dr. Dean Ornish's Program for Reversing Heart Disease*.

How can sprouts play a role in supporting a healthy lifestyle?
Sprouts have a germinative energy that we don't yet have the capacity in science to measure, but I believe this energy is one of the reasons seeds and nuts in general have been shown to be so powerful in preventing and treating so many diseases. Like seeds and nuts, sprouts, by nature, are designed to burst into a plant, and as such, they have benefits above and beyond the nutrients they provide.

What are some of the standouts in terms of nutritional value?

We all know that if you eat broccoli, it's great. If you eat broccoli sprouts, it's even better. A 2011 study from the University of Illinois found that combining broccoli with broccoli sprouts actually might increase the anticancer effects that each has on its own. A team at Johns Hopkins found that a daily serving of broccoli sprouts for two months reduced the marker for the presence of H. pylori, the bacteria that can lead to ulcers and gastritis, by 40 percent.

Do you think it's feasible for patients to adopt a sprouting lifestyle?

In and of themselves, sprouts are relatively inexpensive, and most of the time it takes them to sprout is not supervised time, so to the extent that people can incorporate sprouting into a busy life, it's to everyone's advantage. And of course, you have the option of buying them at the grocery store.

Can sprouts be useful in food deserts?

Back in 2000, I worked with the CEO of McDonald's to put salads on the menu. McDonald's has millions of customers a day, and many of them live in food deserts where there are no grocery stores. The idea was that putting a healthy item on the menu would give people a choice. But what I hadn't realized was that the salad would be priced at $5.99 while the burger was 99 cents. So if you were on a fixed income, you'd get more calories for your dollar by eating junk food, though of course it doesn't factor in the real cost of the food in terms of subsequent health care. Sprouting could offer an affordable source of produce to food deserts.

How do sprouts compare with vitamin supplements?

A number of studies have shown that vitamins don't necessarily decrease the risk for chronic disease, and in some cases, they even increase it. For example, studies show that when vitamin A was given to smokers, it actually increased their risk of lung cancer. Whereas when you get your nutrients from food, there are almost uniformly beneficial effects. With that food, you are also getting literally tens of thousands, if not hundreds of thousands, of other protective substances, such as phytochemicals, bioflavonoids, carotenoids, retinoids, and isoflavones to help reduce the risk of many chronic diseases. Sprouting can only make those effects more beneficial. So with few exceptions, it's always better to get your nutrition the way it comes in nature rather than through a pill.

SUPER SPROUTS

A Seismic Shift in Nutrition
with the Healthiest Food
on the Planet

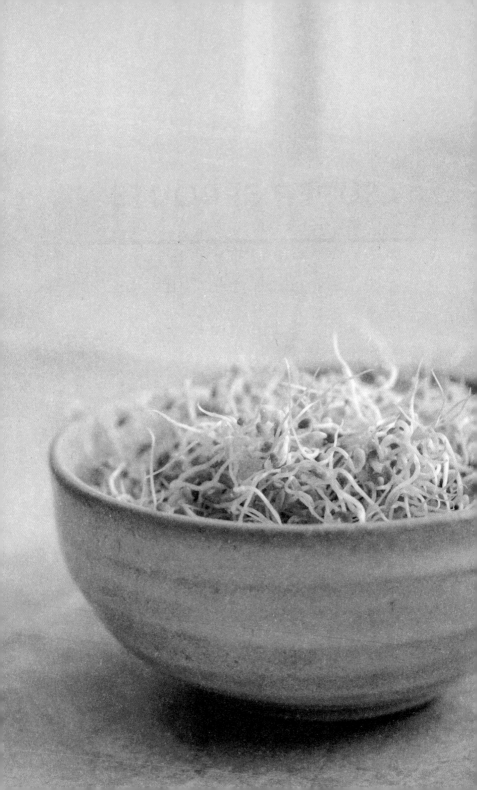

THERE'S ONE THING people of every dietary persuasion can agree on: We need to eat more plants. Most of us are deficient in the nutrients plants contain but are daunted by current dietary advice to fill our plates with mostly plants. Who has the time?

Enter sprouts: Sprouts are the most efficient delivery system for the heroic amounts of veggies we need to eat to maintain or regain our health. In fact, there is literally no food on earth more nutritious than sprouts. Everyone can sprout, and an increasingly wide variety of sprouts—from the standard mung to punchy onion sprouts and broccoli sprouts containing ten to one hundred times the cancer-fighting compounds of mature broccoli—are becoming readily available at natural food stores and supermarkets. I believe that there is no downside to eating sprouts, and the medical doctors and nutritionists I have spoken to all support the consumption of sprouts. Sprouts are an ancient food, but they have just what our bodies are craving today.

Sprouts are inexpensive and have the potential to feed the world, enabling us to eat locally in any season and increasing the reach of real food in food deserts for millions of people. Toss sprouts with dressing and you have an instant super salad with no chopping or special prep needed. But there is so much more you can do with sprouts. The recipes in this book—from sprouted hummus to low-sugar, protein-filled sprout smoothies, soups, and wraps—show how easily sprouts can upgrade our daily meals. Sprouts are the next frontier in food!

Sprouts multiply like weeds, but they are complete vegetables in and of themselves. For example, three tablespoons of broccoli seeds will grow in physical volume about ten times in under a week to about two cups of fully edible and super-nutritious plants. What's also amazing is that you don't need to be an expert gardener or even an experienced sprouter to get started. All you need are seeds and some basic tools you might already have around the house. They don't even require soil or sunlight.

Nature's First Food

Each living organism, from red delicious apple to tropical mango, garden rose to prairie grain, begins as a seed. The blueprint for the biological development and function of the plant is contained in the small seed and remains the same from seed to sprout.

Imagine a lion in the savanna stalking its prey or a herd of zebras along the horizon. While this carnivore has its place in nature, our story centers on the herbivore and frugivore. Grazing the grasslands, the gazelle ingests green growth its entire life, receiving the complete spectrum of nutrients it needs. As humans, we can take a hint from this herbivore's health habits.

How do we integrate more green grass and green vegetables into our lives and the lives of people we love? By starting with the seed, nature's first food. Seeds, and their resulting sprouts, roots, shoots, and leaves, are nothing new. Almost all plants require seeds to reproduce, and human animals and wild animals have been consuming seeds since the beginning of time.

In my early sprouting days, I thought of sprouts as alfalfa, mung bean, broccoli, clover, and sunflower. I never put two and two together to conceptualize that all plants start as seeds, and all seeds can sprout, shoot, and root and turn into microgreens and then full-blown plants. It was a revelation to me. I had a whole new world of nature to dig into, no pun intended. I am absolutely fascinated by seeds, and I hope that when you learn about them and add a little love to turn them into food, you will be too.

SEEDS ARE A TREASURE

Seeds are at the heart of the nutrition in fruit. One of the things that excites me the most about eating fruit is collecting the seeds and sprouting them. The expression that one man's trash is another man's treasure couldn't be more applicable to fruit seeds. If you were to go online to buy citrus seeds, you would pay fifteen cents or more for each seed, and as much as four dollars per seed for exotic citrus like the giant pomelo. That's more than the fruit itself, which would contain many seeds.

Most people eat the creamy green flesh of the avocado and throw out the seed. Guess what? The avocado seed, a.k.a. the *pit*, is one of the best sources of soluble fiber available and is extremely rich in antioxidants and the mineral potassium. As a matter of fact, more than half of all the antioxidants in an avocado come from the seed. To get at the nutrition of the avocado seed, rinse the pit and soak it in water overnight. Insert three or four toothpicks into the sides of the pit and suspend it in a small glass of drinking water with the larger bottom half in the water. Keep replenishing the water for two to three weeks, until you see the seed start to sprout, then crack it open and add it to the blender (you'll need a high-speed blender) when you're making a smoothie. The taste of an avocado seed is bitter, but it will be well masked by the other ingredients in your smoothie.

A few years ago, I was carving open a butternut squash. After meticulously peeling the pale orange beast, I cut it in half to find dozens and dozens of sprouted squash seeds. The shells looked like pumpkin seeds, but the sprouts looked like mung bean sprouts. I ate every one of them.

Considering that I eat about a half ton of produce a year, you could appreciate how much I love fruit. But out of all the everyday and exotic fruit I've ever enjoyed, my favorite is watermelon with seeds. I remember sharing slices of watermelon on a date and watching my new friend pick out the watermelon seeds and feeling sad that she was missing out on the full richness of the experience. It's becoming harder and harder to find organic watermelon with seeds, but when I do, I buy as much as I can carry and store. Hopefully, this sends a message to the retailer to request more. It gives me so much pleasure to eat an entire meal of just watermelon with the seeds. Give it a try—you'll love it and feel great.

I hope the point that seeds are valuable is coming through! I'll leave you with one more fun one: sprouting a coconut. Start with a green or brown coconut from your yard (or most likely the market) that has no visible signs of rotting. The coconut should have water inside when you shake it. Soak

it in a bucket of drinking water for three days. Add rocks
or bricks to a clay or plastic three- to five-gallon (ten- to
twelve-inch-tall) pot with drainage holes at the bottom, then
fill it with organic potting soil. Bury the bottom two-thirds
of the coconut, leaving the stem or top area out of the soil.
Store indoors in a warm room—at least 68°F. Remember
that coconuts come from the desert or the tropics. Water
it frequently to keep the soil moist, and avoid all-day direct
sunlight. Keep at it for two to six weeks, until you see a six- to
twelve-inch green leaf that looks like a baby palm tree growing
out of it. A magical kind of fusion occurs between the coconut
meat and water to expand and fill the entire shell. To open
it, you smash it with a hammer or meat cleaver. Then you
get to eat everything inside it. It tastes like mature coconut,
but fluffy and lighter. Imagine a cross between coconut and
cotton candy. It's a delicacy worthy of sharing on a special
occasion.

MULTIPLYING BY THE MILLIONS!

Nature has created complete infinite systems for plants to
thrive on the planet. The earth would survive fine without
humans, but not without seeds. Seeds, when given the right
amount of love, will grow and multiply a thousandfold, a
millionfold, or more.

This is not just poetic. Take the acorn, for example. Acorns
have not been cultivated for consumption in America, but
wildlife have eaten them in various ways over time. A clear
indication that an acorn is edible for humans is when it's
sprouting! Otherwise, it has potentially poisonous tannins and
antinutrients, designed to protect it to grow into more oak
trees. A single acorn can grow into an oak tree, and an oak

tree can produce as many as ten thousand acorns in a season. The white oak tree has an average life span of three hundred years with recordings of trees as old as six hundred years. The back-of-the-envelope math says that 1 oak tree = 3,000,000 acorns (i.e., 10,000 acorns/year × 300 years), and that's not including the acorns that go on to grow into oak trees and produce more acorns. And a single sunflower can contain between one and two thousand sproutable seeds. The power of plants and seeds to multiply is simply astounding.

From Seed to Sprout

Plants contain six major parts: the stem, leaf, flower, root, fruit, and seed. The seed could easily be mistaken for a pebble, a speck of dirt, or even a piece of wood. But what's inside a seed is nothing short of miraculous. The seed is the giver of life for the plant.

A seed is an organ of the plant. In technical terms, in the case of flowering plants known as the *dicots* (such as pea, broccoli, and peach), it's the reproductive organ of the angiosperm. It's a structure that's formed by the maturation of the ovule within the ovary of the angiosperm, the mature ovule.

The seed is comprised of several parts. These include the seed coat, which is derived from the maternal tissue of the ovule. It's like the armor for a knight—it protects the inner parts of the seed from freezing, excessive heat, and being broken under pressure and water. The seed coat can be hard, thick, or thin and either light or dark. The outer part of the seed coat is called the *testa,* and the inner part is called the *tegmen.* The seed embryo is the part of the seed that hosts the roots, stem, and leaves.

When you add water to a seed, you ignite it to begin the germination process.

After a plant is fertilized, the male and female gametes form a zygote. This is a combined cell that can grow and divide itself and then grow into a new organism. The zygote eventually will form the plant embryo, which is protected by the plant coat. It also develops its endosperm, which is the food the plant will consume during the early stages of germination. And this is the food that we as humans get to eat too when we sprout seeds.

Sprouting a seed is relatively simple, and if you create the right environment and you are using high-quality, high-germination seeds, you are most certain to activate the dormant seed and create a highly active, fast-growing sprout. The right environment includes water, lighting, temperature, and type of vessel. During the early stages of growth, the seeds are relying on the energy of a chemical fuel called *adenosine triphosphate,* or *ATP.* ATP acts as the carrier of energy in all living organisms from humans to mushrooms. ATP uses the energy that is released from the explosion of nutrients and makes it available to the reactions that need that energy, such as growing a seed into a sprout. ATP will carry the seed through its early stages until the sprout forms leaves and begins making its own food through photosynthesis.

The seed will rely on the endosperm for food and the ATP for energy until the miniature leaves, actually the cotyledons, are formed and they start producing chlorophyll. Chlorophyll's molecules convert the energy of the sun to carbon dioxide, carbohydrates, and oxygen. This process is called *photosynthesis.* The sprouting process is like a massive birthing process for the seed happening on a submicroscopic level.

The seed could remain dormant for lifetimes, or, when placed in the right environment and when water is added to it, the sprouting process begins. To follow the play-by-play journey of seed to sprout, choose your method from Your Sprout Garden (pages 107–164) and watch the miracle of nature's first food in action. Now let's learn about all the many reasons to sprout, from the joy of sprouting to the health that comes as a result.

DR. ALAN GOLDHAMER: "THE OPPOSITE OF EMPTY CALORIES"

Alan Goldhamer, D.C., is the cofounder of TrueNorth Health Center, the largest facility in the world specializing in medically supervised water fasting and an exclusively plant-food diet free of added salt, oil, and sugar. Sprouts are an integral part of the protocol at TrueNorth, where more than twenty thousand people have regained their health over the past thirty-five years.

What are your top three reasons to sprout?

1. *Sprouts are an inexpensive source of high-nutrient, low-caloric-density food. All you need is pure water, high-germination seeds, and a container with a screen.*
2. *Sprouts are a ready source of fresh whole foods. They can be grown easily anywhere on the planet at any time. Think of sprouting as plant fortification—a great way to get in your greens out of season.*
3. *Sprouts taste great!*

Who should sprout?

Sprouting is limited to people who don't want to be fat, sick, or miserable. People looking to add diversity of flavor and texture to their food will also enjoy sprouting. Do you want to have organic food all year round? Sprouts are the answer.

When were you first turned on to sprouts?

I worked in a health food store when I was sixteen, and soon after, I started a sprout company called Perfect Sprouts, which put me through chiropractic school. Perfect Sprouts was one of the first businesses to introduce sprout mixes, such as mung, lentil, adzuki, and pea. We would grow two thousand pounds a day! We worked a lot with restaurants, because lettuce is seasonal, expensive, and requires processing, but a handful of sprouts costs dramatically less, leaves no waste, and adds heft to sandwiches.

What are you sprouting at TrueNorth?

Our goal is to add as much whole food into people's diets as we can, and sprouts not only add nutrition, they change up the flavor. Our favorites are pea, sunflower, buckwheat, lentil, and clover, and we like to throw in some spicy mustard, radish, and fenugreek sprouts for added flavor. Each has its own nutritional profile.

What is your recommended daily protocol for sprouts?

It depends on where you live and the season. When you don't have access to fresh produce, you should sprout more. But a variety of sprouts, preferably that you grow yourself, is an excellent addition to your diet all year round. Consider sprouts a form of supplementation without taking a pill—sprouts are basically all nutrients with few calories. A huge salad with sprouts and other fiber-filled greens will satisfy you without overloading your system. It's the opposite of empty calories!

So Many Reasons to Sprout

Sprouting has been around since the beginning of time on this earth. The nutrition in a handful of sprouts is the same if not more than the nutrition of the whole plant. Think about how efficient this is. The following are some of my favorite reasons to sprout.

Easy: Everyone can learn to sprout, and kids can even join in. It feels magical, but there is no actual magic involved. It's nature at its best. Sprouting requires basic equipment, water, and seeds and just a few minutes a day. You can literally use things you already have in your kitchen or garage, such as glasses, jars, strainers, and colanders. Turn to page 107 to learn how to sprout.

Fast: Gardening is intimidating to many people. It's a lot of work up front with relatively little yield in terms of flowers, greens, or edibles. Growing leafy greens or fruits can take weeks, months, a whole season. On the other hand, sprouting is so simple and the results are back so quickly that they're practically growing right in your face, making it easy to keep a steady supply going in your kitchen. The small seeds, the grains, the salad seeds, and even the legumes become edible in as soon as two to three days. Broccoli sprouts hit peak nutrition for sulforaphane on the third day. At any given time in my kitchen, I could be sprouting a dozen different seeds in trays, automatic sprouters, jars, and bags. My routine for watering, rinsing, straining, and spraying all those sprouts can be completed from start to finish in as little as five minutes.

Low cost: Organic food, in particular fresh organic vegetables, can be expensive. Depending on where you purchase them, baby lettuces can cost between sixteen and twenty-four dollars per pound. Fresh sprouts that you grow on your own cost significantly less than half of that. You can buy organic seeds for as little as seven dollars per pound, and they will multiply in size by as little as four times and as much as ten times. If you do the math, even with the most modest estimates, we are talking about fresh, ripe, organic vegetables for under two dollars per pound. That would make a four-ounce serving of sprouts cost under fifty cents. This data makes me want to shout from the rooftops and stop people on the street to share the good word with them! It's really incredible how much edible, nutritious, plant-based food comes from a small number of low-cost seeds.

Local: *Very* local. Most produce travels hundreds of miles and, in many cases, thousands of miles before it makes its way onto your plate. Aside from the environmental impact and the fossil fuel costs of transportation, consider freshness. On average, it takes about one week for produce to get picked, packed, sent through a distributor and to a retail store and then to the shelf before it's purchased and brought home. With sprouting, you sprout it, you eat it when it's sprouted. You can't get fresher than that.

Plant-based: The research about the benefits of a whole-food, plant-based diet is abundant. There are dedicated books, movies, websites, seminars, retreats, conventions, and courses. Some of the top athletes in all fields happily and enthusiastically recommend a whole-food, plant-based diet based on the personal benefits they have experienced. There probably are more plant-based books on Amazon today than there were total books in the first month the site first launched back in 1994. It's plain and simple: whole fruits, vegetables, seeds, nuts, and seaweeds are more nutritious on a per-calorie basis than animal products. Almost every doctor and governing agency will agree that we all should be eating more fruits and vegetables. The U.S. Dietary guidelines recommend eating seven to thirteen servings of fruits and vegetables every day. This makes the argument for sprouts very easy because they are incredibly and exponentially more nutritious than their mature counterparts. A wide array of sprouts would contain practically every single vitamin, mineral, micronutrient, phytonutrient, antioxidant, polyphenol, bioflavonoid, and so on that we need.

Fun: The best chefs find their passion working with their hands to create what they believe is healthy food to feed other people and themselves. What makes it fun is engaging all the senses in the process. The more you get comfortable with sprouting, the more fun it will be and the better results you will have. I get such a kick out of connecting with nature by using my hands, my head, and my heart to create edible food from dry seeds. And kids will find it fun without even thinking about why!

Anticancer: The research on the cancer-fighting content of sprouts is compelling. Read about it on pages 46–47.

Delicious: I find sprouts to be so tasty that I crave them constantly. Because of my obsession with sprouts, I am constantly sharing them with just about everyone I encounter, and I can usually find a few varieties that any given person will like or love off the bat. It might take time to fall in love with sprouts on their own, but the good thing is that you don't have to eat them plain like a cow grazing on grass. That's where the recipes on pages 165–229 will make a sprout fanatic out of you!

Digestible: If you think about the fact that your body is mostly comprised of water, it makes sense that the higher the water content of the food you consume, the easier it is to digest. Every sprout is different, but what all sprouts have in common is that they are at least 50 percent water. It takes twenty-four to seventy-two hours for the body to break down a four-ounce piece of steak, chicken, or fish, while a four-ounce serving of sprouts takes as little as one hour. If you chew the sprouts well, your teeth are acting as the juicer, blender, or masticator, breaking them down into smaller particles that are easily digestible and enriched with micronutrients, soluble fiber, insoluble fiber, amino acids, and a tad of fat. In the last few years, there has been a lot of discussion about the lectins, an antinutrient, legumes contain. But wait, aren't there so many good reasons to eat legumes? My answer is a resounding yes. Eat them, but soak and sprout them first. The lectins exist in the legume to protect it, and the secret to reducing the lectins to make the legumes more bioavailable and more digestible is sprouting.

Empowering: Sprouts help you control your food destiny. The simplest sprouting protocol is to soak the seeds overnight, rinse them twice a day, and then eat the sprouts. Seeds have a very long shelf life, are very easy to store, and take up very little space. Knowing how to sprout and having a store of seeds makes me feel truly empowered. There are many days when I eat sprouts and nothing else, and those days I stand up straight, my energy is high, and I feel strong. Eating an abundance of sprouts keeps me satisfied but not stuffed. I marvel at the nutrition that I am consuming and know that I am doing something really, really good for myself.

Good for the air: There have been studies by highly respected institutions like NASA, Pennsylvania State University, and the University of Georgia to name a few that suggest plants clean the air inside the home. Sprouted seeds, in the form of microgreens like basil, celery, and sunflower shoots, get exposed to light and start to grow green leaves as they mature. The leaves on the plants have pores, which absorb gases. The research indicates that plants can absorb carbon dioxide, benzene, formaldehyde, and other volatile organic compounds. That means that plants may help remove hidden toxins in cleaning products, plastics, fabrics, carpets, cosmetics, and cigarette smoke and overall upgrade the air you breathe.

Sustainable: One of the greatest lessons in reducing waste comes from Burning Man, the largest "leave no trace" event in the world. Seventy thousand people create a temporary city in the Nevada desert over the course of a week. Absolutely everything you bring into Burning Man must be taken out with you. When you don't have a garbage disposal or trash can nearby, you see how quickly trash, packaging, and food waste adds up. On the other hand, repurposing trays, jars, bottles, and baskets as a major means of creating food is very exciting for me. My plan for the next Burn is to feast on sprouts. I'll simply bring a few glass jars with seeds and jars and colanders to sprout in. One relatively small bag will contain enough dry seeds for me to sprout for the whole week and leave no waste, no compost, no plastic. From past experience with sprout feasts, I know that I will thrive there eating sprouts!

Great conversation starter: In my days of the grind and hustle, I was monomaniacally focused on work and didn't like to socialize. Now that I am sprouting, I love to share the information, and people are—pun intended—eating it up. Those new to sprouting generally are mesmerized, and people already into health and nutrition want to go deeper. Everyone resolves to find a way to add more sprouts to their lives.

Educational for children: In the United States and in particular cities, many families grow up without a garden or ever visiting a farm. They think that food comes from the grocery store or, if they are lucky, an organic co-op or natural food store. Sprouting at home is a wonderful opportunity to bring nature into the house and show, tell, and eat sprouts. Kids love it!

Diet-friendly: Sprouts are an incredibly nutritious food with only a fraction of the calories of other foods. That makes them amazing for people who like to eat! Weight Watchers considers all fruits and non-starchy vegetables zero points on their system. Even though beans and peas are pretty carb-heavy, they also have a lot of naturally occurring fiber and are filling and delicious, so Weight Watchers encourages you to eat them. Incidentally, most vegetable sprouts fit into most diet plans, from Paleo to Keto, Atkins, low carb, and high carb.

KALE CAN'T HOLD A CANDLE TO SPROUTS

It seems as though kale came out of nowhere, hit its peak, and has stabilized as a fixture in healthy diets across the board. According to the Department of Agriculture, farmers produced 50 percent more kale in 2012 than they did back in 2007 with more than twenty-five hundred farms harvesting kale in 2012. By 2014, Whole Foods Market was selling twenty-two thousand bunches of kale per day in its stores. That's more than sixty bunches per day per store. I loved kale way before Beyoncé wore a kale shirt, but the facts show that kale doesn't hold a candle to sprouts. If you compare mature kale to sunflower, buckwheat, or broccoli sprouts, it's practically a nonstarter from a nutrition perspective. The sprouts will have an average of twenty-five times the nutrition of mature kale— or any other mature common green leafy vegetables, for that matter. Don't get me wrong, kale has got a lot going for it, especially if you spend two months growing it so that you can have it fresh from your garden, but sprouts beat kale when it comes to nutrition, accessibility, price, convenience, and variety. In nature, animals don't just eat one plant. Gorillas eat around 142 different types! Can we even name that many vegetables? Enjoy the full menu of sprouts that nature offers at a fraction of the cost of that bunch of kale at the market.

EVERY SPROUT IS A POWERHOUSE

A comprehensive study by a researcher at William Paterson University in New Jersey published by the Centers for Disease Control and Prevention came up with a list of forty-one "Powerhouse Fruits and Vegetables" ranked by the amounts of the seventeen critical nutrients that they contain. Powerhouse fruits and vegetables are defined as being most strongly associated with reduced chronic disease risk and containing 10 percent or more daily value per 100 kcal of seventeen qualifying nutrients (potassium, fiber, protein, calcium, iron, thiamin, riboflavin, niacin, folate, zinc, and vitamins A, B_6, B_{12}, C, D, E, and K). Guess what? Every single one of those forty-one has seeds that can be sprouted and eaten. (FYI, the top ten are watercress, Chinese cabbage, chard, beet greens, spinach, chicory, leaf lettuce, parsley, romaine lettuce, and collard greens.)

HOW TO EAT SPROUTS

1. Look, stare, *gaze* at your sprouts for at least one minute. This may sound a little woo-woo, but it's anything but; taking a pause to connect with your food is the beginning of the digestive process and will psychologically and physiologically prepare your body for what you're about to eat.
2. Eat your sprouts slowly and deliberately. Connect with their flavor and freshness, and enjoy every bite. Many people tell me they are shocked by how delicious sprouts are. Don't miss out! Find out which ones you like the most, and soon you'll know what you are in the mood for.

3. Avoid cooking your sprouts. They have a high water content, and when they are heated, they will wilt away and may lose their flavor, texture, and aesthetic—and in some cases, their nutrients. The rare sprout, notably the mung bean sprout in its mature form, is hearty and tough enough to withstand a hot soup or even a little stir-fry.

DR. JOEL FUHRMAN: "A GREAT ADDITION TO ANY DIET"

Dr. Joel Fuhrman, M.D., six-time *New York Times* bestselling author and writer of the foreword to this book, and internationally recognized expert on nutrition and natural healing, is best known for coining the term *Nutritarian*, which refers to a plant-rich, longevity-promoting way of eating that favors foods with a relatively high proportion of nutrients to calories. That means lots of vegetables, including sprouts!

What makes sprouts so healthful?
In their earliest stage of development, plants produce more phytochemicals, which fight off insects and other natural predators. As plants grow and get hardier, they lose some of those protective phytochemicals. As sprouts are essentially plants when they are young, eating sprouts gives you the highest concentration of phytochemicals and anticancer compounds—for example, there are much higher levels of sulforaphane in broccoli sprouts than there are in broccoli florets, stems, and leaves.

In addition to broccoli sprouts, which other sprouts do you recommend?

There has been a lot of research on broccoli sprouts, but if we took kohlrabi sprouts, mustard green sprouts, or kale sprouts, we'd probably get similar results. It's always to our advantage to eat a diverse range of foods for optimal nutrition. Sprouted foods have nutritional spectrums that are different from those of their mature counterparts, adding that all-important variety to your diet.

How do you serve sprouts at your health retreats?

We like to combine sprouts and other vegetables in our salads for bulk, chewiness, and extra fiber. Adding sprouts to salads increases their concentration of anticancer nutrients, and when you toss them with a nut- or seed-based dressing, you further increase the absorption of the phytochemicals. In doing so, you maximize the quality and digestibility of already healthy foods. You can turn a bean into a vegetable to make bean sprouts, and you instantly increase the micronutrients in the food you're eating. Some of the sprouts we also like to use at the retreats include radish sprouts, clover sprouts, and pea shoots.

Who should eat sprouts?

Sprouts are a great addition to any diet: They are easy to make, and they make eating organic food more affordable and accessible.

Sprouts as a Nutritional Supplement

From as early as I can remember growing up, I always took a multivitamin. Or at least I was supposed to. I remember everything

from GNC, to Flintstones chewables, to generic mystery tablets. For whatever defiant or intuitive reasons, I usually would
hide them and rarely chewed or swallowed them. When I first
became plant-based, a.k.a. vegan, I heard so much about what's
missing in the diet that I needed to supplement.

Now the research is out on some synthetic vitamins used
for supplementation, and it's surprising and encouraging. *Not*
encouraging to take synthetic vitamins but encouraging to
eat a plant-based diet with lots of sprouts. For example, vitamin B_9 can be derived from folate, which occurs naturally in
plants, or from the synthetic form, folic acid. Our bodies can
absorb folate through digestion, but our bodies don't convert
folic acid into active B_9 very well. And supplementing with
synthetic beta-carotene can do a person more harm than good
(see pages 34–35). ConsumerLab tested a number of multi-
vitamins and found problems in almost half, with a number
of products containing either much less or much more of the
nutrients listed. The gummy vitamins many parents earnestly
feed their kids were some of the worst offenders—80 percent
of them failed their testing. I'm all for taking our cue from
the federal government's 2015–2020 Dietary Guidelines for
Americans: that our nutritional needs should be met primarily from foods. That said, if you aren't getting regular
direct sunlight, then, vegan or not, it could be a good idea
to supplement with vitamin D (the current RDA is 600 IU
daily), and it is recommended that vegans supplement with vitamin B_{12}, typically with drops under the tongue or a sublin-
gual tablet.

The following is a sample of the targeted nutrition sprouts
can supply.

Sulforaphane

Sulforaphane is a phytochemical that is naturally found in many plants, in particular cruciferous vegetables like asparagus, bok choy, broccoli, cabbage, cauliflower, and kale. Within the cruciferous vegetables, there is both myrosinase (an enzyme) and glucoraphanin (a glucosinolate). When cruciferous vegetables are chewed, the enzyme myrosinase transforms glucoraphanin into sulforaphane. Studies have shown that raw broccoli has ten times the amount of sulforaphane as cooked broccoli, and additional studies have shown that broccoli sprouts have five to ten times the amount of sulforaphane as raw broccoli.

Population studies have linked a higher intake of eating cruciferous vegetables like broccoli with a significantly reduced risk of cancer. They believe that the compound sulforaphane is in part responsible for the anticancer properties.

In vitro testing has demonstrated that sulforaphane has properties that have anticancer effects on both the size and the quantity of various types of cancer cells. This is not new information. The *New York Times* broke this story back in 1997, and the testing continues. There has been good news across the entire cancer spectrum relative to sulforaphane in breast cancer, prostate cancer, colon cancer, skin cancer, bladder cancer, throat cancer, and lung cancer. Sulforaphane may release antioxidant and detoxification enzymes that protect against cancer.

In both test-tube and animal studies, sulforaphane has shown that it may benefit the human heart by reducing inflammation, which is linked to clogging of the arteries and high blood pressure. Sulforaphane was shown to reduce fasting blood sugar levels by more than 6 percent and to improve hemoglobin A1c (an indication of blood sugar levels over the previous two to three months). The tests had the most impact on participants who were at high risk from being obese or having poor diabetes control. Sulforaphane has also been shown effective for people living with autism (see page 43) and Alzheimer's disease (see page 44) and those who have sustained brain damage (see pages 42–43). It also has been shown to help counter constipation (see page 44) and protect against sun damage (see pages 44–45).

Sulforaphane appears to accomplish some of its powerful healing effects through epigenetics, the relatively new discovery of how changes to diet and lifestyle can make genetic changes. This is how we instruct cells to turn on and off, and sulforaphane has demonstrated the ability to influence the part of the DNA that affects diseases.

Beta-Carotene

There have been a lot of studies on dietary intake of beta-carotene from fruits and vegetables, including an extensive analysis in the *Journal of the National Cancer Institute*, associating it with lower risk of breast cancer and other long-term benefits. This logically would encourage some people to run out to the store to buy a beta-carotene supplement. But what the world didn't realize at the time was the mortal danger that came with ingesting synthetic beta-carotene, which is created from isolated fragments of vitamins and may be made from benzene extracted from acetylene gas.

A peer-reviewed, double-blind, placebo-controlled study published in *The New England Journal of Medicine* gave over twenty-nine thousand male smokers beta-carotene and vitamin E to assess their cancer-protective benefits. The researchers found out that there was a significantly high incidence of lung cancer (close to 20 percent) in those consuming the beta-carotene supplement. To make matters worse, the mortality rate was 8 percent higher among the participants of the study who received the synthetic supplement.

There are many fruits and vegetables that have beta-carotene, including carrots, sweet potatoes, dark green leafy vegetables, squash, cantaloupe, red and yellow bell peppers, apricots, peas, and broccoli. We don't need to supplement with synthetics to get what we need. In fact, the University of Maryland and the USDA did a comprehensive analysis of the nutrient composition of twenty-five sprouts and microgreens and found that practically across the board, the leaves had considerably higher nutritional densities than their mature counterparts.

Omega-3 Fatty Acids

Open a search window, type *omega-3,* and you will get more than five hundred million results. This is one of the nutrients that has been studied quite extensively over the last two decades. I suspect that may be because of the huge market for fish and fish oil supplements. Americans now consume more than one hundred thousand tons of fish oil every year. Fortunately for us, we get to benefit from that research and bypass the fish products to get it. By the way, where do you think the fish get the omega-3s in the first place? They get it from algae.

Omega-3s are the fatty acids that you definitely want to have in your diet, and you can get an abundance of them from plants, seeds, nuts, and, you guessed it, sprouts. Many of us know about the role of omega-3s in heart health, including lowering triglycerides and blood pressure and raising HDL (good) cholesterol, and preventing blood clots and plaque from forming in our arteries. Omega-3s can help manage insulin resistance, thereby reducing the risk of adult-onset diabetes. They reduce inflammation, the root of many diseases. Omega-3 fatty acids are important parts of the membranes that surround the cells in the human body. One study demonstrated the effectiveness of omega-3s as adjuvant therapy in treating patients with colorectal cancer.

What's more, studies show that people who suffer from depression improve when they consume more omega-3s. Omega-3s are critically important for pregnant mothers because the developing infant needs them for brain health and growth. There is research that focuses on ensuring that a baby gets enough omega-3s during the first year to lessen the risk of autoimmune diseases, including diabetes, autoimmune diabetes, and multiple sclerosis. There are studies that observe a reduction of symptoms, including improving attention span and task completion for children with ADHD. They also can be effective in decreasing hyperactivity, impulsiveness, restlessness, and aggression. (Wait a moment while I go tear into my Chia Pet.)

Not surprisingly, omega-3s can be effective in the treatment of lupus, arthritis, colitis, Crohn's disease, and psoriasis. What aren't they good for! The top seeds to sprout for your hit of omega-3 fatty acids are chia seeds, flaxseeds, and hemp seeds. Sprouting helps remove the enzyme inhibitors from the seeds and makes the omega-3s more bioavailable. (Note: Walnuts are another excellent source of omega-3 fatty acids; they don't sprout, but you can unlock their nutrition by soaking them before you eat them.)

Protein

Barely a day goes by when someone who finds out I am plant-based doesn't ask me the inevitable question, *Where do you get your protein?* I used to get annoyed, look them straight in the eye, and tell them that I was "taking the Fifth." As the years have gone by, sometimes I'll answer, *Where does a bonobo get its protein?* When the person inevitably tells me I'm not a bonobo, I'll explain that my DNA is pretty darn close to a bonobo's, and bonobos are largely vegetarian. They are fast enough and strong enough to command most animals in the jungle, and they are predominantly plant eaters. Why? Is it because they don't watch TV? It's my instinct that they are connected to instinct and intuition, and they are guided to eat plants.

I've never met someone with a protein deficiency who didn't have anorexia, bulimia, or another disorder, but obesity is very real, and so are diabetes and heart disease. That said, protein is very important to the human diet for everything from building muscles to keeping depression away, and sprouts have plenty of protein in a low-fat, low-calorie, and easily digestible form. Standouts include sprouted lentil, chickpea, almond, alfalfa, broccoli, pea, mung bean, and clover, and soybean and quinoa sprouts are complete proteins. A green pea–rich smoothie will fuel you with protein more efficiently than processed pea protein powder—what a great way to start the day!

Vitamin C

Vitamin C is one of the vitamins that must be consumed through food or supplementation, as the body can't produce it on its own. Vitamin C is a strong antioxidant that boosts the immune system by protecting cells from free radicals; free radicals are dangerous because they can create oxidative stress, which has been linked to many chronic diseases. Vitamin C is anti-inflammatory and increases blood antioxidant levels by up to 30 percent. Vitamin C comes predominantly from fruits, vegetables, and, not surprisingly, sprouts.

A little bit of vitamin C magic happens when you sprout. Some dry seeds, such as lentils, have 0 percent of the RDI (Reference Daily Intake) of vitamin C, but sprouted lentils have 14 percent! Soybean, mung bean, pea, alfalfa, and broccoli sprouts all have vitamin C in them, with broccoli sprouts containing 23 percent of the RDI in a single cup. Note that vitamin C is very sensitive to heat and degrades considerably with cooking, which is one of many good reasons to eat your sprouts uncooked.

Folate

Folate is the naturally occurring, water-soluble form of vitamin B_9, and it's often confused with folic acid, which is synthetic. In 1998, the U.S. Food and Drug Administration began mandating manufacturers to enrich breads, cereals, flours, cornmeal, pasta, rice, and other grain products with folic acid to reduce the risk of neural tube defects. Folate has many important roles in human nutrition and is particularly important for women who are contemplating having a baby and men who are planning on being fathers.

Folate is found in many sprouts, including legume sprouts, asparagus sprouts, arugula sprouts, and, no surprise, broccoli sprouts. The content of total folates in broccoli sprouts increases twenty-four-fold during the first eight days of germination.

Iron

Iron carries oxygen in the hemoglobin of red blood cells throughout the body to produce energy and remove carbon dioxide. It's not fun when your iron levels become low; you could experience unpleasant side effects like fatigue, headaches, dizziness, and pale skin.

There are two types of iron: heme and nonheme. Heme iron is found only in meat, poultry, and seafood (this form is not required for the body). Nonheme iron is found in plant-based foods like grains, beans, vegetables, fruits, nuts, and seeds. Nonheme iron is also found in eggs and dairy. Sprouted legumes, lentils, soybeans, chickpeas, peas, quinoa, hemp seeds, flaxseeds, and sesame seeds are great sources of nonheme iron. So eat your sprouts, and make sprouted nuts and seeds your go-to snack to be strong like Popeye!

Vitamin K

Vitamin K refers to the fat-soluble vitamins K_1 and K_2. These vitamins play a role in blood clotting and regulate bone metabolism and blood and calcium levels. Vitamin K comes from many different fruits, vegetables, and sprouts. Vitamin K is found in almost all sprouts, in particular green salad sprouts and legumes.

Among the top K legumes and nuts you can sprout are green peas, soybeans, and mung beans, and vegetables like kale, mustard greens, swiss chard, collard greens, beet greens, parsley, spinach, broccoli, brussels sprouts, and cabbage. And this one is a showstopper—one cup of watercress contains 106 percent of the RDI of vitamin K!

Fiber

All plants have fiber, and no animal products have fiber. There are literally zero grams of fiber in meat, chicken, fish, or cheese. It comes as no surprise, then, that most people in the United States fall short of the recommended daily intake of between twenty-five and thirty-eight grams of fiber.

Sprouts to the rescue! Sprouts contain both soluble and insoluble fiber. Soluble fiber is credited for reducing the risk of heart disease by lowering LDL cholesterol and by balancing blood sugar levels. Insoluble fiber, a.k.a. dietary fiber, isn't digested, but it does move things through your system. Sprouts can help you with your overall digestion because when seeds are sprouted, their fiber increases and becomes more bioavailable, countering constipation and resulting in great poops.

DR. JOEL KAHN: "SPROUTS ARE THE NEW APPLE A DAY"

Joel Kahn, M.D., is one of the world's top cardiologists and a bestselling author. It is his belief that plant-based nutrition is the most powerful source of preventative medicine. He champions food as medicine and has devoted his career to educating others about the healing power of plants. One day, he wants to drive a car powered by sprouts, called the Alfalfa Romeo.

What is your relationship to sprouts?

I've been following a plant-based diet for forty-two years, and I've been a sprout addict for the past fifteen years. One of my three kids did a formal ten-week health course at Hippocrates Health Institute, and I spent a fair amount of time with him there. The daily protocol that we enjoyed would always include sprouts. I love broccoli sprouts, but all sprouts are nutritionally powerful. At GreenSpace Café, my plant-based restaurant in metro Detroit, just about every plate, from salad to lasagna to chili, goes out with fresh organic sprouts on top. We have a producer that uses a hoop farm to provide fresh sprouts twelve months of the year.

From your perspective as a cardiologist, do you see any downside to eating sprouts?

Sometimes you get them between your teeth, but nothing worse than that! When anyone asks me about a particular food, my question is: What would you be eating otherwise? *Sprouts are an instant dietary diet upgrade, in particular for those eating the standard American diet, but also for some of the better eaters who are still falling short on their intake of nutritionally dense, alive, and healing foods. There isn't a diet in America that wouldn't be better with a serving of sprouts. Sprouts are the new apple a day.*

What is your ideal sprout protocol?

Start the day with a freshly pressed green juice including sprouts, have a salad that's bigger than your head and totally cover it with sprouts, and end the day with a small cooked-food meal with sprouts as an accoutrement. I recommend pea protein powder as a supplement for some of my patients, but sprouts would be a step up in nutrition whenever possible. Grow your own sprouts at home if you can, and liberally add them to any dish.

Sprouts for Targeted Health

The concentrated nutrition in sprouts makes them potent medicine and a powerful companion to whatever healing program you may be participating in. Much of the research is in its beginning stages, but what we have already is incredible.

Brain Health

Sprouts contain massive amounts of nutrition that can help the brain function at optimum levels. Cruciferous sprouts like broccoli and radish contain sulforaphane, which stimulates the expression of the cytoprotective genes (genes that are protective of the cells) in the brain. Ongoing nutrigenomic research is revealing a deeper understanding of these chemical reactions, adding to the compelling data connecting plant-based nutrition and brain health. Sulforaphane activates the central nervous system and suppresses inflammation. A study investigated whether the administration of sulforaphane would ameliorate two behavioral functions, and it did by reducing inflammation safely. This study was performed on rats, but it has significant implications for the treatment of brain damage and is inspiring more testing.

Broccoli, cabbage, pea, soybean, and lentil sprouts are rich in manganese, a trace mineral that is essential for the development of nerve and brain functions.

Autism

The latest science indicates that the most effective treatment for autism may be sulforaphane from broccoli sprouts. In an eighteen-week study of forty autistic boys and men, more than half of the patients in the study improved in their social interaction, verbal communication, and behavior. Researchers noticed that the sulforaphane created some of the same effects as fever on the subjects in the study. The theory is that sulforaphane treatment may trigger a biological reaction called the *heat-shock response* that eases the symptoms of autism. The preliminary data indicated that 31 percent responded positively at fifteen weeks.

In another study, seventeen of twenty-six participants who were administered sulforaphane showed noticeable improvements in behavior, social interaction, and calmness, in particular improvements on the Social Responsiveness Scale, while given treatment. Most of all the improvements disappeared after the treatment, further supporting the results of the study.

There is now a patented, pharmaceutical-grade product used for testing the effects of sulforaphane. From my perspective, broccoli sprouts are the bona fide source and that testing should be done with both. It should be noted that Johns Hopkins University is both a stockholder of and is entitled to royalties from a sulforaphane supplement.

Alzheimer's Disease

Efforts to find a means of treatment for this neurodegenerative disease are ongoing. Sulforaphane has been put to the test, and one study concluded that "sulforaphane can ameliorate neurobehavioral deficits by reducing cholinergic neuron loss (the neurons located in the basal forebrain) in the brains of mice with Alzheimer's disease. The mechanism by which it works may be associated with neurogenesis (the development of nerves, nervous tissue, or the nervous system) and aluminum load reduction." This is very early research, but the potential of sulforaphane to be used in Alzheimer's disease therapeutics is exciting.

Constipation

It is well known that following a whole-food, plant-based diet gives us the fiber needed to alleviate or eliminate constipation. This fact was taken to a whole new scientific level when one scientist tested and concluded that the daily consumption of broccoli sprouts could normalize bowel movements in healthy subjects. He studied the impact of sulforaphane on reducing chronic oxidative stress (the imbalance between free radicals and antioxidants), which can impact bowel movements, by measuring how sulforaphane affects gut bacteria.

Sun Damage

Sulforaphane mobilizes cellular defenses that protect skin against damage by ultraviolet radiation. Ultraviolet radiation can cause

DNA damage, inflammation, and suppression of the immune system. It can also lead to nonmelanoma and melanoma skin cancer. Scientists tested a topical application of sulforaphane-rich extracts of three-day-old broccoli sprouts, and they found it protected against inflammation and edema and reduced susceptibility to erythema (redness of the skin).

They also tested sulforaphane as a dietary component, and it provided powerful protection against a wide variety of damage that occurred by exposure to ultraviolet radiation from the sun, and its effects were clearly evident two to three days after treatment. This long-lasting property has not been demonstrated by topical sunscreens.

Cardiovascular Health

Cardiovascular disease is the number-one killer of women and men in the United States. Fortunately, the science says that there is hope. There is a lot of research about plant-based diets reversing, arresting, or preventing heart disease. I believe that there is now more than enough information to attest to the benefits of a *true* plant-based diet for cardiovascular health (Oreos are vegan, and so is Coca-Cola, but I wouldn't recommend them).

Sprouts are an easy decision when it comes to matters of the heart. Overall, sprouts can help lower cholesterol, reduce inflammation, and slow the formation of plaque to prevent heart disease. Chia seeds have the highest amount of omega-3 fatty acids of not only all sprouts but all plant-based food. Hemp seeds and flaxseeds also contain a fair share of omega-3s. The American Heart Association recommends three servings of grains a day; those could easily and affordably be sprouted grains.

All nuts contain healthy fats, which have been shown to prevent arrhythmias and reduce the risk of developing blood clots. According to the Mayo Clinic, nuts can lower blood levels of low-density lipoprotein to help prevent heart disease. While not all nuts and seeds can be sprouted, they all can be taken to the soaking stage, which makes them more digestible and their nutrients more accessible.

Cancer Prevention

According to researchers at Johns Hopkins University School of Medicine in Baltimore, broccoli sprouts contain between thirty and fifty times the concentration of cancer-protective chemicals found in mature broccoli. These naturally occurring chemicals exist not only in broccoli but other cruciferous vegetables, including horseradish, kale, collard greens, cabbage, brussels sprouts, cauliflower, bok choy, mizuna, turnip root greens, napa cabbage, rutabaga, mustard seeds, arugula, watercress, radish, daikon, and wasabi. Every single one of those vegetables starts out as a seed and therefore can be sprouted. Specifically, cruciferous vegetables contain glucosinolates, which are under research for their potential in targeting some types of cancers. The research on their anticancer impact has gone so far as to see a major pharmaceutical company trying to patent sulforaphane. It's such a hot topic in the medical community that specific, peer-reviewed research is getting into the weeds and exploring which sprout has the most bioavailable anticancer compounds. But the most important thing to know is that cruciferous sprouts fight cancer and are incredibly easy to incorporate into your diet.

DR. JOSEPH MERCOLA: "I EAT SPROUTS DAILY IN MY SALADS"

Joseph Mercola, D.O., has had the most visited natural health website in the world for the last fifteen years, Mercola.com, dedicated to providing up-to-date natural health information and resources. Dr. Mercola is the author of several *New York Times* bestselling books and is also famous for his daily sprout-centered salad.

When did you first get turned on to sprouting?
About eight or nine years ago when I first visited Hippocrates Health Institute here in Florida. They had dozens of different sprouts growing, and they taught me how to grow the ones I was most interested in. I learned that as living, nutrient-dense food, sprouts have a lot of benefits, and they're easy and relatively inexpensive to grow.

Have you encountered any difficulties in sprouting?
If you don't do it right, you may have a problem. In Florida, it's pretty warm, and sprouts like a temperature of about 70 degrees. When the temperature in the room gets much below that—into the 50s and 60s—you might not see as much growth. And in humid environments, you might encounter mold if you're not diligent in cleaning your trays; this could devastate your crop. But in my experience, I haven't encountered any problems at all—I find sprouting to be very easy.

Which are your favorite sprouts?

I primarily use sunflower shoots, but I'm also a real fan of broccoli sprouts and cauliflower sprouts, primarily because of their potent phytochemicals, in particular sulforaphane, which has some magnificent properties I'm very fond of.

Do you think other sprouts can rival broccoli sprouts if there were more research?

Absolutely. Sulforaphane is one of the most studied glucosinolates, but there are dozens of others. It takes decades to understand the complex biochemistry that's going on and then for the research to get out there.

How often do you eat sprouts?

Most every day, usually as part of a salad. Instead of lettuce, I'll typically start with about a cup of sunflower shoots as my primary green and sometimes clip some wild fennel greens and add them in. Other veggies I include are shredded carrots and sometimes bell pepper, and I'll dress the salad with some of my organic blueberry apple cider vinegar.

Skin Care

It's not a surprise that eating a whole-food, plant-based diet with a lot of fresh sprouts will make your skin glow. Sprouts have antioxidants, which kill free radicals from the sun and environmental pollution and protect the skin from sun damage and skin cancer. Pea sprouts contain vitamin B, which helps healthy skin development. You can make a pea sprout compress by juicing pea sprouts; apply it to your skin to hydrate and tone it.

The vitamin C in sprouts helps produce collagen, which provides elasticity to your skin and can promote faster healing. The sprouts that contain omega-3 fatty acids, most notably chia, hemp, and flax, can help reduce inflammation and reduce or reverse acne and other skin problems. Fenugreek sprouts have a naturally occurring silica; silica is required to rebuild and regenerate the skin's connective tissues. Fenugreek sprouts can also remove toxins from the blood that cause dull skin.

Weight Loss

The most obvious reason to consume sprouts for weight loss is that their high fiber will make you feel full, and their low calorie count means you don't have to count calories. They are rich in many vitamins, minerals, bioflavonoids, antioxidants, and omega-3 fatty acids. The more sprouts you eat, the more weight you will lose, as long as you stick to a whole-food, plant-based diet. It's an all-around victory.

Autoimmune Disease

Autoimmune diseases occur when the immune system attacks the cells in the body. Doctors aren't sure of all the triggers of autoimmune diseases. Autoimmune diseases have similar symptoms like joint pain, joint swelling, inflammation, fatigue, and weakness. It is thought that the gut may play a significant role in the immune system because it's predominantly housed there. A whole-food, plant-based diet is a gut-friendly diet, and it automatically omits some of the top inflammatory offenders, such as dairy and refined sugar. Adding plentiful sprouts to the mix is one of the best next steps you can take to keep inflammation at bay.

SPROUTING FOR PETS

If you had told me twenty years ago to feed my dogs sprouts, I would have looked at you like you were crazy. Even after being vegan for more than fifteen years, the thought never crossed my mind. Now that I have upped my sprouting capabilities and always have sprouts around, I feed them to hungry dogs. Guess what? They love them. Generally, dogs and cats like foods that they can sink their teeth into and chew, so the crunchy bean and legume sprouts, soybean sprouts, and sunflower sprouts tend to be met with approval. To find out your pets' favorites, hand-feed them some sprouts and see what they like and love. If they don't eat them out of hand, it's easy to start to mix a small percentage into their normal feed and then build up over time.

Almost all cats and dogs like sprouts, but don't be alarmed if they throw them up sometimes. Sunflower sprouts can be a better option, as they are easier to swallow and digest. If you grow your sprouts in a tray, try leaving the tray by your pet's bowl for a few hours during the day for them to grab a snack, then place it out of reach, although dogs and cats generally won't overeat sprouts.

SPROUTING IN FOOD DESERTS

People living in food deserts don't have much of a choice whether or not to eat healthfully. TV, radio, and print advertising glamorizes, sensationalizes, and unethically seduces people to eat unhealthy products, and those are the products you'll find in abundance there.

As programs like the Edible Schoolyard continue to grow, plant-based education in the schools will become more commonplace. And similar to how urban gardens are opening up new avenues to fresh fruits and veggies, I can easily see sprouting clubs forming around the country, with bulk buying of seeds and swapping recipes and information. Active, successful sprouters could share their knowledge to bring serious nourishment to food deserts. Because sprouts are so nutritious and inexpensive to grow, they can be an answer to fresh produce for everyone, everywhere.

DR. JOSH AXE: "SPROUTS ARE ONE OF THE MOST NUTRIENT-DENSE FOODS IN THE WORLD"

Josh Axe, D.C., D.N.M., C.N.S., is a doctor of chiropractic, certified doctor of natural medicine, and clinical nutritionist with one of the most renowned functional medicine clinics in the world. He is the founder of the website DrAxe.com, which is one of the top natural health websites in the world, covering topics of nutrition, natural medicine, fitness, and recipes. He is also the author of several bestselling books.

When did you first realize there was something special about sprouts?
Years ago, when my mother was diagnosed with cancer. I researched ways she could heal her body, and I put together a natural health

protocol incorporating several diets with anticancer properties, including Gerson therapy and the keto diet. This meant drinking vegetable juices, eating high-fat foods, cutting out sugar, and incorporating healing herbs and spices like turmeric and ginger into her diet. I had her eating a lot of salads containing sprouts, in particular broccoli and clover sprouts, as had I learned that sprouts are one of the most nutrient-dense foods in the world. Mom is now in her midsixties and cancer-free.

Are there any sprouts in particular that you would recommend?

The two I consume the most are broccoli sprouts and mung bean sprouts. I love that broccoli sprouts are very high in vitamin C and anticancer sulforaphane. In traditional Chinese medicine, mung bean sprouts are considered a nutrient-dense food and are highly recommended for cooling heat in the body and reducing inflammation. They also are high in vitamin C and are a really good source of fiber and protein. When I'm making a salad for myself, I like to add broccoli sprouts and mung bean sprouts as a base and often throw in clover or another sprout for variety.

What's the difference between taking a vitamin C supplement and consuming sprouts such as mung that are naturally high in vitamin C?

To best absorb certain nutrients, you need other nutrients with them; it's a synergistic relationship. For example, vitamin C works best with quercetin and bioflavonoids. You're going to the whole package in a whole food like sprouts rather than taking a vitamin C supplement. Food sources are always most effective.

Do you have concerns about the safety of sprouts?
I recommend seeking out organic sprouts, which are even better if they're from a small grower. It's rare for organic produce to have food safety issues.

You talk about freshness and sustainability in your book *Eat Dirt*. What role do sprouts play?
You're never going to get anything fresher and more sustainable than eating food you grow yourself. There are studies that show that the nutrient value of produce goes down substantially every day after harvesting, so I'm a big fan of consuming food when it's most alive and nutrient rich. The longer a living food sits on a supermarket shelf, the more nutrients will be lost. The fresher the better!

A SPROUT PRIMER

From Adzuki to Broccoli,
Chia, Mung, Mustard, Onion,
Radish, Sunflower, and More

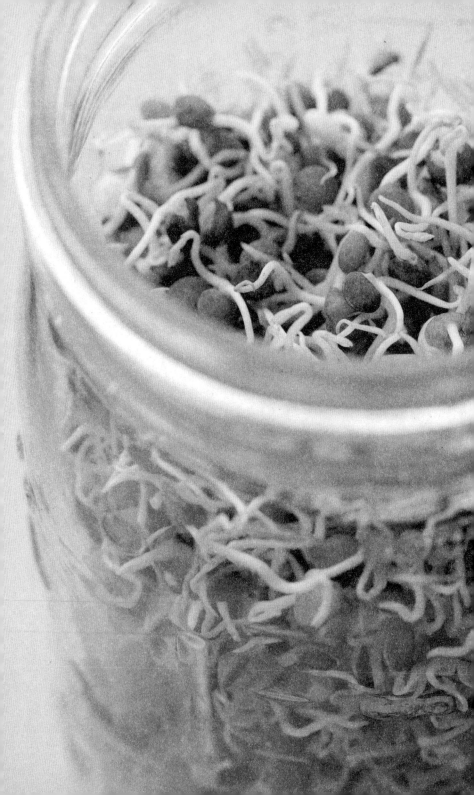

PEOPLE OFTEN ASK me what my favorite sprout is. To me, that's like asking a parent who their favorite child is. I love each sprout equally for its unique taste, texture, and benefits. Each and every sprout has something unique to offer, and I hope the facts, figures, and stories I'm about to share with you will compel you to try them all! Categories to choose from are Salad Green Sprouts (page 59), Legume and Bean Sprouts (page 80), Shoots (page 92), Grasses (page 95), and Grains, Nuts, and Seeds (pages 99–101). See pages 102–105 for a quick-reference how-to sprouting chart.

I very much believe in Dr. Joel Fuhrman's philosophy of "eat to live" (versus "living to stuff your face with food that's designed and engineered to make you addicted"). From my own personal experience, I will give you an idea of what makes each individual sprout unique and what to expect when you eat them.

Note of caution: Sprouts—in particular, alfalfa sprouts—are a raw agricultural product and may contain harmful bacteria and have been linked to serious injury and death. Pregnant women, infants, children, the elderly, and persons with lowered resistance to disease have the highest risk of harm, which includes bloody diarrhea, vomiting, fever, dehydration, hemolytic uremic syndrome, Guillain-Barré syndrome, reactive arthritis, irritable bowel syndrome, miscarriage, or death.

This is a very real warning, and it should be taken seriously. If this book was about meat, chicken, fish, dairy, I would be writing a very different and strident warning. As with all things, you must be careful, do your homework, and make decisions that you feel comfortable with.

Sprouts, Shoots, and Microgreens

A *sprout* is a shoot of a plant, a new growth from a germinating seed. It's a broad definition that encompasses every plant included in this primer, including shoots and microgreens, but there are some specifics that define the latter two.

Shoots literally shoot out of a seed with the intention of going above ground. They begin at the earliest stages of germination. Technically, all sprouts have shoots that come out of the seed. As the plant matures, the shoots grow into stems and leaves, making them part of the shoot system. The shoot system is what drives the growth to gain access to the light and convert that light energy into the chemical energy of sugar. Learn about sunflower shoots on pages 93–94 and pea shoots on page 93.

Microgreens are seedlings that are harvested before they develop into larger plants, like sprouts that have gone the extra mile. Consider them a nutritionally dense version of the mature plant. Arugula, basil, beet, kale, and cilantro microgreens have become the garnish of choice for elite chefs. People talk about microgreens like they haven't been around forever, yet they are simply a relatively new label for a mature sprout or immature plant. In the following section, I call out basil and celery to be grown specifically as microgreens, as they are difficult to fully sprout, but just about any vegetable seed that can germinate can continue to grow into a microgreen. Microgreens can be grown in either soil, a growing medium, or unbleached paper towel with great success.

Salad Green Sprouts

The choices are many, from the standard alfalfa, broccoli, and clover you'll find in stores, to the lesser-known sprouts, such as basil, watercress, and fenugreek that I invite you to sprout at home. Salad seeds are easy to sprout—most can grow in glass jars (pages 127–130) and trays (pages 140–143), and even sprouting bags (pages 133–137) with a little care. Some, like the most playful of sprouts, chia, are gelatinous and require a different (but easier!) setup that I go into on pages 132–133. Just about any seed can be sprouted; the following are just a sampling of the more common salad sprouts. Peruse through a seed catalog (see Resources, pages 233–234) to take in the range of what's available.

Salad sprouts have become so much a part of my daily salads that I rarely eat mature greens anymore. You could literally replace all the greens in a Caesar salad, chopped salad (see the house sprout salad on page 204), or any other salad, or at a minimum add them to supplement the greens already there to spike the nutrition, freshness, and flavor. Then you have freshly harvested salad greens all four seasons!

Alfalfa Sprouts

This most common sprout was immortalized as hippie food in Woody Allen's 1977 film *Annie Hall* when Allen's character, Alvy, tries to act hip at an LA vegetarian restaurant by placing an order for "alfalfa sprouts and a plate of mashed yeast." But the hippies knew a thing or two about food, and we have the movement to thank for today's veggie-forward focus and the current availability of alfalfa sprouts in natural food stores and supermarkets across the country.

Alfalfa the crop actually goes way back; it was first cultivated in Persia more than six thousand years ago, where it was known as the "father of all foods." The mature alfalfa plant is bitter and needs to be cooked and seasoned to enjoy it. But the raw alfalfa sprout is mild in taste and full of nutrition in its natural state.

Alfalfa sprouts are rich in phytoestrogens that naturally mimic human estrogen. There have been many studies that indicate they can reduce the risk of breast cancer. They can also help relieve symptoms of menopause like mood swings.

Alfalfa sprouts have a mild flavor, almost like shredded romaine lettuce, and are crispy. They take to other flavors and seasonings well and don't try to compete. Eat them in a sandwich or smoothie or as a salad topper, or just grab a handful and eat as a snack on the go.

Note: Alfalfa sprouts contain an amino acid called *L-canavanine* that may increase inflammation in people with lupus by stimulating the immune system. As a result, people with lupus and similar autoimmune conditions are advised to avoid alfalfa sprouts completely. To reduce the risk from

L-canavanine, alfalfa sprouts should be eaten on days 7–10, after they have become more developed. It has been reported that the L-canavanine peaks on the third day and decreases daily. L-canavanine can also be reduced by rinsing the alfalfa sprouts twice daily (which you will be doing with all your sprouts), as L-canavanine is water soluble.

Although alfalfa sprouts are wildly popular, they also have been targeted by mainstream media, which continues to ignore the benefits of fresh food and their relatively small risks (see page 247). I always use USDA organic alfalfa seeds (preferably seeds that have been laboratory tested for human pathogens), wash them with a sanitizing agent (see page 124), and keep them cold. In my twenty-five years of sprouting, I have never had a problem, nor have I heard of anyone who has had a problem sprouting at home. That being said, it is up to you to make your own informed decision.

Arugula Sprouts

Rocket is what they call arugula in the UK. I guess it's because of the unique shape of its leaves, but I like to think it's also because of the kick of spice it has. Arugula sprouts are gelatinous, which makes them hard to sprout commercially. But at home, it's very easy because you get to skip over the soaking and draining most sprouts require. And their peppery flavor gives a unique, sophisticated taste profile to anything you add them to.

Arugula is a member of the brassica family of greens that includes radishes, kale, broccoli, and cabbage, making them as much a superfood as any others out there. Most of the research has been on the mature arugula plant, but fortunately, we can lean on a University of Maryland study that educates us on how much more potent and nutritious microgreens are than their mature counterparts. Arugula is jam-packed with micronutrients and macronutrients—I think of the concentrated nutrition in the sprouts as a multivitamin containing vitamins A, C, K, and B$_2$, folate, and a bountiful number of minerals, including potassium, calcium, magnesium, and phosphorus as well as the antioxidant beta-carotene.

Use arugula sprouts as a sandwich topper or garnish or mixed in a salad with milder sprouts to balance their bold flavor.

Basil Microgreens

Basil, also known as St. Joseph's Wort, is a green herb that is part of the mint family. It's originally native to tropical regions of Asia, where it was grown specifically for medicinal uses. Basil has been making headlines for its plethora of nutrition, and growing basil sprouts gives you a unique combination of health benefits and culinary delight.

When germinated, basil seeds are an anticlimactic sprout. The small brown seed will sprout a tiny white tail. But if you wait and continue to water, rinse, or spray, you will be able to nurture your basil into a microgreen, a nutritionally dense version of the mature plant. I like to harvest them at the one- to two-inch stage. Grow basil microgreens using the same method as growing sunflower shoots in soil (see page 153), extending their growing time by a few days.

TIP: *Juicing basil microgreens in a wheatgrass auger juicer will produce a very intense concentrated juice like wheatgrass. It takes a handful of basil microgreens to yield a 1-ounce shot of basil juice. You can drink it straight or use an eyedropper to infuse any food with concentrated basil flavor. Consume immediately, or add garlic or fresh lemon or lime juice to keep it fresh for a few hours.*

The mature basil plant is considered to be antiaging, antibacterial, and anti-inflammatory. I haven't found specific data on basil sprouts or microgreens, but if you consider that one cup of fresh basil leaves has over 10,000 mg of vitamin A, or 350 percent of the recommended daily allowance, and that microgreens by nature contain higher concentrations of nutrients than the fully grown plant, one can only imagine the exponential increase in nutrition you get from the younger version of the greens! It may come as a surprise that, weight for weight, basil has almost as much potassium as bananas, and I would guess that basil sprouts and microgreens have even more! "Basil is rich in polyphenols that drive gut health and general good health by reducing oxidation and inflammation," says Barry Sears, Ph.D., a leading research scientist in the field of inflammation.

Basil microgreens have a similar taste profile to the mature herb and therefore can be used interchangeably. They are so tender that even a little heat will permanently damage them. They play nicely with other herbs like oregano, summer savory, rosemary, and sage, and nothing beats them as a topper for in-season sliced tomatoes. Basil microgreens ground with raw pine nuts make the absolute best and most nutritious pesto. I am warning you—once you taste it, it will be gone before you even have time to grab a cracker or crudités!

KATIE WELLS: "SPROUTING ENABLES FAMILIES TO CONNECT WITH THEIR FOOD"

Katie Wells has a background in journalism and is a mom of six. She is the founder of the wildly popular website Wellness Mama, with more than fifteen hundred blog posts to its credit. She is also the author of three books and has been named one of the one hundred most influential people in health and wellness. Her family are avid sprouters, and she often writes about the benefits of sprouting in her blog.

What inspired you to start writing about sprouts in your blog?
My background is in journalism, so I spent a good amount of time reading studies on sprouts before I started writing. The research on sulforaphane in broccoli sprouts in particular stood out. I was inspired to write about the subject because sprouting is an easy plant-based practice anyone could do right in their kitchen, and it's ideal for urban moms who don't have the space for a garden. It's a way for families to have a connection with their food, and that connection lends itself to conscious eating.

Which sprouts do you typically have growing?
I pretty much have broccoli sprouts growing all the time. I have Hashimoto's thyroiditis, and eating broccoli sprouts is part of the protocol for keeping the nodules from growing. I'll also rotate in other sprouts, such as alfalfa sprouts.

How receptive has your mama audience been to sprouts?

There are some small vocal segments that are worried about food safety. Those are the mamas who are still using antibacterial soaps; I do the most educating with them to open them up to the bigger picture. But most mamas realize sprouting is a good thing; some are aspirational, while many are starting to realize the benefits of sprouting at home.

How do you incorporate sprouts into your family's diet?

Sprouts make it into about half of our meals, whether it's in a salad or wrap or even just a topping. I usually add a bunch to my smoothies. I personally will consume up to two cups of broccoli sprouts a day.

How do your six kids feel about sprouts?

I started them on sprouts pretty young, so they are used to the taste and have no problem eating them.

What are your top reasons to sprout?

1. ***Sprouts add variety.*** *Our diets have changed, especially in the last hundred years. We used to consume two hundred plants or so on a regular basis, and now it's five for most people. Sprouts add variety and important micronutrients to our vegetable rotation.*

2. ***Sprouts are budget-friendly.*** *Budget is a concern for most moms. Growing your own sprouts costs a fraction of what you would pay at the store.*

3. ***Sprouts connect us with our food.*** *From a mom's perspective, it's important to see where our food comes from. Our kids should know that food doesn't always come from the grocery store.*

4. ***Sprouts reduce waste.*** *Sprouting is a way to grow food at home sustainably, with minimal to no packaging.*

5. ***Sprouts are really good for you.*** *Sprouts can even be prescriptive for certain conditions. For example, when I got diagnosed with Hashimoto's thyroiditis, one of the things the doctor recommended was a small amount of broccoli sprouts every day to keep down the tumor activity of the disease.*

Broccoli Sprouts

In the 1990s, broccoli sprouts took the main stage, and for very good reasons. While sprouting in the United States became popular among the "crunchy hippies" in the 1970s, the discovery of sulforaphane and glucoraphanin created the first global seed shortage of broccoli seeds. There are more than one thousand published studies that have identified sulforaphane as one of the most potent food-derived molecules ever discovered.

What has hit the news is their anticancer abilities; broccoli sprouts have been shown to kill cancer stem cells and slow tumor growth and are helpful in regulating and activating more than two hundred different genes. What's also amazing is the bioavailability of the sulforaphane in broccoli sprouts. According to the research, about 80 percent of what's ingested finds its way into the body's cells. Read about the role of broccoli sprouts in cancer care and prevention on pages 46–47.

What's just as remarkable is that with all the drugs and all the research, the most effective treatment for autism may be sulforaphane from broccoli sprouts. Read more about that on page 43.

Chewing, cutting, grinding, and perhaps even juicing broccoli sprouts allows the enzyme myrosinase to come into contact with glucoraphanin. When these two substances come in contact, a chemical reaction is triggered wherein the myrosinase converts the glucoraphanin to an isothiocyanate, sulforaphane, the superhero substance that broccoli sprouts have become famous for. Note: The research shows that three-day-old broccoli sprouts consistently contain ten to one hundred times the amount of glucoraphanin found in mature broccoli. At three days is the ideal time to harvest, rinse, and store broccoli sprouts.

The best way to eat broccoli sprouts is to add them to everything! They have a little kick to them, which I love. If your tastes run mild, their bite will easily get lost with almost any dressing or sauce. Eat them by the handful, juice them in a wheatgrass juicer, add them to smoothies (page 172), blend them into pesto (page 219) . . . eat them all day long!

BROCCOLI SPROUT DETOX

The anticancer properties of cruciferous vegetables, including broccoli and broccoli sprouts, is widely known. What's new news is that broccoli sprouts can detoxify pollutants. People throughout the world are breathing polluted air, and it's now proven that broccoli sprout powder can boost the defense mechanism that accelerates the rate at which the body clears pollutants so that less harm is evoked by them.

A study by scientists from Johns Hopkins School of Public Health successfully tested a broccoli sprout beverage. In the study, they took three hundred women and men and gave them a beverage concoction with and without broccoli sprout powder. Blood and urine tests showed the control group with broccoli sprout powder had a 61 percent increase in the excretion of benzene and a 23 percent increase in the excretion of acrolein, both carcinogens. The test involved broccoli sprout powder, so I can only imagine what the results would look like if they had used fresh broccoli sprout juice or just a healthy amount of broccoli sprouts!

Cabbage Sprouts

In its mature form, cabbage looks almost like iceberg lettuce but is miles above in nutrition, as it's actually part of the cancer-fighting cruciferous family in which broccoli and cauliflower belong. Cabbage sprouts are a miniature but potent version of the mature vegetable, and you can easily sprout green or red cabbage seeds.

Green cabbage sprouts contain more folate than red cabbage, and red cabbage sprouts contain bonus anthocyanins, an antioxidant that gives red, purple, and blue foods their color. I believe that the beauty of these antioxidants is to visually attract us to eat them and reap their rewards. And red cabbage sprouts will reward us in many ways. For starters, they contain forty times more vitamin E and six times more vitamin C than mature cabbage. They are loaded with amino acids and, in particular, L-glutamine, which is great for your digestion. There is even research indicating that red cabbage sprouts can help with cancer prevention, antiaging, eye health, and reducing inflammation in the gastrointestinal tract.

Cabbage sprouts are crunchy and taste mild and sweet like

cabbage, making them easy to eat. You can eat them alone as a snack or as an addition to any meal. Try adding them to cereal for you or your kids for an interesting texture and flavor addition. They work well with other veggies to create a sprout-centered Buddha bowl. You could even ferment them in the way you would make sauerkraut, which would make them a "force multiplier" by adding probiotic benefits to an already powerful food.

A 2016 study published in the *Journal of Agricultural and Food Chemistry* showed that red cabbage microgreens can lower circulating LDL cholesterol in mice fed a high-fat diet. This shows promise for humans, as heart disease is the leading cause of death in the United States and high cholesterol is a major risk factor. The data indicates that microgreens can control weight gain and cholesterol metabolism and may protect against heart disease by preventing high cholesterol in the blood.

Celery Microgreens

Celery sprouts are not for the impatient sprouter. They take a long time compared to broccoli or even sunflower shoots. At some point, you may actually think that they are dead and will be tempted to throw them out. Seven to ten days can pass before they show any growth, even the slightest, tiniest tail. If you're up for the challenge, go for it, but for our purposes here, I recommend going the microgreen route. Celery microgreens will get you a hearty yield.

Today, celery is all the rage, mostly in the form of celery juice. Mature celery, celery sprouts, and celery microgreens all contain large amounts of potassium (one cup of celery sprouts is under twenty calories and has about half the potassium as one cup of banana, but with 10 percent of the calories and one-fourteenth the sugar), dietary fiber, vitamins A, B, C, and E, iron, magnesium, phosphorus, calcium, zinc, chlorophyll, amino acids, and antioxidants. It's no wonder people are consuming more celery these days. What's surprising to me is that the world hasn't really discovered celery microgreens. I visited more than a dozen health food stores and supermarkets and was unable to find them. So I encourage you to grow your own, because if celery is a nutritional magic bullet, imagine the good celery microgreens are capable of!

Celery microgreens taste very clean and light and have a high sodium content. They are less bitter than the leaves of mature celery, but you can clearly identify that they are in the same family. They can be added as a garnish to a soup or salad. If you have enough of them, you can enjoy them all by themselves with a little seasoning or, as I do, unadorned.

THE BEST CELERY JUICE YOU COULD EVER IMAGINE

You can juice celery microgreens in a wheatgrass juicer for arguably the best celery juice you could ever imagine. It's so intense that all you need is a tablespoon, and that's probably all that you will get from a batch of celery microgreens. This may feel anticlimactic since it's going to take you two weeks for less than a serving size of cough medicine. I suggest that you wait until you are in a flow of making many different sprouts simultaneously so you can enjoy the tiny bounty of celery sprouts as part of your overall sprouting routine.

Chia Sprouts

Chia sprouts are the most fun of all sprouts to play with and to eat, à la the Chia Pet. But don't let that fool you. Chia is serious nutrition, and the little seed is said to have been used by Maya and Aztec cultures for supernatural powers. The first record of chia comes from the Aztecs as early as 3500 B.C.; it was one of the primary foods in their diet. *Chia* means strength to the Maya; this was the food that the warriors and athletes ate.

Chia is a versatile seed and can be eaten in many ways— raw, soaked, ground into flour, added to drinks, even pressed into oil, and, of course, sprouted. One ounce packs 138 calories, 9 grams of the good fats that we need, 10 grams of fiber, 5 grams of protein, and 18 percent of the daily value of calcium. Chia and their sprouts are very low in calories and very high in nutrition. They contain higher levels of ALA omega-3 fatty acids than salmon, without the added mercury.

Chia sprouts are fast and easy to grow. You can actually grow them on almost any surface. Since they are gelatinous, you don't soak them, and you don't need soil; you just keep them moist and they will grow into a very satisfying sprout. (If you were to soak the seeds, you'd wind up something closer to chia pudding, the popular dessert form of this superfood.)

Like most sprouts, chia sprouts can be eaten plain or added to salads or wraps. Try them as an alternative to cilantro in guacamole.

Clover Sprouts

Red clover sprouts should be called *red clover medicine.* They are simply amazing. It has been reported that dozens of cultures around the world use these sprouts as a treatment for cancer. Red clover contains genistein, an anticancer compound that can prevent new blood vessels from forming within a tumor. Since tumors rely on new blood vessels to grow, genistein works to starve the cancer. Red clover sprouts also contain a phyto-estrogen that is similar to the estrogen found in humans. Many women eat them to help deal with the symptoms of PMS, hot flashes, menopause, and even fibrocystic disease.

As with most sprouts, they are low in calories and high in protein and fiber. They also are high in calcium, iron, vitamin C, and folate. A simple 3½-ounce serving contains 38 percent of the RDA of vitamin K, which is paramount for the absorption of calcium and a variety of other minerals, including iron, phosphorus, zinc, selenium, and magnesium.

Red clover sprouts are very easy to eat. They have a gentle flavor and are slightly crunchy. They can be eaten by the handful as a snack and included in salads, soups, sandwiches, bowls, or virtually anywhere on anything! They can easily become invisible and unnoticed in foods you add them to. If you think you don't care for sprouts, blend clover sprouts into a smoothie and you'll get all their benefits without detecting their presence. Or try them in a sprouty take on the garlicky, herby Middle Eastern sauce chermoula (page 218).

Fenugreek Sprouts

Interesting fact: Fenugreek seed is not actually a seed but a legume. Documentation for the use of fenugreek goes back to Egypt in 1500 B.C., where it was historically used to ease childbirth and increase breast milk flow. In contemporary Egypt, women use it to relieve menstrual cramps. Fenugreek has a long history in Ayurvedic texts as well as in Greek and Latin pharmacopoeia. In the beginning, it was revered for its power both as an aphrodisiac and as medicine. Modern-day Ayurveda seems to focus the use of fenugreek more on digestive and respiratory issues. Research shows that by consuming fenugreek, you can stimulate the production of insulin in the body to counteract elevated sugar levels in the blood. This is incredible news for people with type 2 diabetes. Fenugreek is also high in iron and protein.

Bitter is a taste that is sorely lacking in our diets, and in this department, fenugreek delivers. Fenugreek seeds are nutty, slightly sweet, but mostly bitter. Until your taste buds are attuned to bitter, fenugreek sprouts work best as a small side dish (try tossing them with tahini and lemon) or as an accent to a dish containing an element of sweet, such as Lemony Cauliflower Salad (pages 200–201).

Flax Sprouts

Flaxseeds have been around since the beginning of civilization and were one of the earliest cultivated crops. They are so nutrient dense that most sources cite their nutrition by the tablespoon rather than the cup. Flax is a gelatinous seed, so it is sprouted without soaking, using the method on pages 132–133.

Flaxseeds are used across the kitchen the way hammers are used on construction sites—in both obvious and creative ways, such as grinding the seeds in a coffee grinder and adding to beverages or breakfasts or soaking them and adding them to a smoothie for body or even as an egg replacement in recipes. The most powerful and miraculous way is to sprout them. Sprouting unleashes their fullest potential, in particular their omega-3 fatty acids, making them an excellent brain food. They also contain ligands, a phytoestrogen that helps balance and deliver the estrogen, which can help women going through menopause. The fiber in flaxseeds and their sprouts will help you feel full, and flax is one of my favorite sources of protein. Flax can help improve immune function, lower cholesterol, and even prevent tumors. Some fun ways to enjoy sprouted flax include adding them to cereal (such as the ones on pages 176 and 177–178), sprinkling on avocado toast, mixing with coconut yogurt, or topping salads.

Hemp Sprouts

Hemp has been cultivated for more than ten thousand years, making it one of the oldest planted crops in the world. It has been used as a source of calories, nutrition, fiber, fabric, and even paper. Hemp has found its way into everything from plastics used in automotive manufacturing to sprouting bags. An article in *Popular Mechanics* magazine back in 1938 stated that there were more than twenty-five thousand uses for the crop. For some reasons beyond speculation, this crop became illegal in the United States, and the trade all but disappeared.

Thank goddess hemp is back. Although hemp originates from the genus *Cannabis,* it's nonpsychoactive. Hemp is by far my favorite plant, and the sprouts are crunchy and chewy with a very nutty flavor. They are 35 percent protein, and a complete protein at that, and they also contain omega-3 fatty acids. For the past twenty years, it was only possible to purchase hulled hemp seeds or unhulled seeds that were roasted. Now I am seeing whole, organic, unhulled hemp seeds, and I am smiling ear to ear. That's because only the unhulled seeds will sprout. In addition to growing hemp as a salad green, it also is fantastic grown in a tray as a microgreen.

Mustard Sprouts

In America, ketchup is the condiment for hamburgers, and mustard is for hot dogs. Considering I haven't eaten a hot dog or even a soy dog in well over a decade, mustard was off my radar. But when I came across mustard seeds, it opened a whole new world for me. Commercial mustard containing large amounts of distilled vinegar is no comparison to the pure hit of mustard flavor the sprouted seeds can deliver. Sprouted mustard seeds are one of the spiciest sprouts available—with a bite akin to wasabi's—and will add a definite kick to soups, salads, and other dishes. Use them sparingly, as a garnish or mixed with other sprouts.

Mustard seeds have been traced back to the time of Hippocrates, when they were used for medicinal purposes. In most cultures that cook with spices, mustard is part of the lineup. Mustard seeds have such compounds as glucosinolates and myrosinase as well as selenium that are known to use phytochemicals to impede the growth of cancer cells. They also contain the nutrients copper, iron, magnesium, and selenium, which can help prevent asthma attacks, regulate blood pressure, and decrease the symptoms of rheumatoid arthritis. They also are a good source of vitamins A, B_6, and C. They belong to the cruciferous family, along with broccoli, so I expect that once mustard sprouts are further studied, we'll be seeing some solid stats on them!

Mustard seeds, both brown and yellow, grow into a wonderful sprout in five to six days, and if you let them grow longer, they will be a delightful microgreen in eleven to fourteen days.

Onion Sprouts

Onion sprouts taste somewhere between onion and scallion, and they look a little like a miniature scallion sprouting from a tiny black seed head. They make a sophisticated swap for scallions and can be grown in just over a week. Onion sprouts are mini powerhouses with high doses of vitamins A, B, C, and E. They contain many minerals, including calcium, iron, magnesium, niacin, phosphorous, potassium, and zinc. You might not think of onions as a source of protein, but onion sprouts are up to 20 percent protein! They also are rich in essential amino acids.

Because they are an intense and concentrated source of nutrients and flavor, you'll do well with small amounts of these special sprouts. Try them in the Tomato and Onion Sprout Soup (pages 181–182).

Radish Sprouts

There are many varieties of radish sprouts, and they all have a real peppery kick. My favorite are daikon radish sprouts, a sharp contrast to the long white root they grow into. The nutrition in radish sprouts is epic. A cup of them has only sixteen calories, less than a sneeze, because they are 90 percent water.

They are also super high in vitamin C and many B vitamins. They have high amounts of folate, which promotes cardiovascular health by breaking down homocysteine, which is thought to promote atherosclerosis.

Broccoli sprouts are today's showstopper sprout, but I suspect that it may be a case of better marketing. My money would go on radish sprouts as top dog. In fact, a little-known 2007 study found that radish sprouts have potentially greater chemoprotective action against carcinogens than broccoli sprouts.

Radish sprouts make a great snack for spice lovers. I can consume an eight-ounce cup in about five minutes if I am present when I chew them, or two minutes when I inhale them. Now that I learned that you really need to chew them to activate them, I stop and chew them like somebody is watching. Radish sprouts can be added to almost anything. Try them blended with kimchi for a creamy vegan cheese dip (page 188).

Watercress Sprouts

Watercress is seldom the first choice of vegetable for consumption in the early twenty-first century; great fame goes to kale, brussels sprouts, and broccoli. My aspiration is to put watercress in the same sentence. That's because watercress sprouts and microgreens are low in calories and high in micronutrient density. *Really* high. According to the Centers for Disease Control and Prevention, watercress is number one on its "Powerhouse Fruits and Vegetables List" with an astounding 100 percent nutrient density. It contains 100 percent of the RDI of vitamin K, which is important for healthy bones and for blood clotting.

One cup of watercress contains more than 20 percent of the

RDI for both vitamin C and vitamin A, plus 106 percent RDI of vitamin K. Watercress is a great source of antioxidants (beta-carotene, zeaxanthin, and lutein) as well. In a recent study, watercress as a whole-food source of these antioxidants outperformed all the other vegetables in the study in its ability to help the body to neutralize free radicals.

Watercress sprouts and microgreens are dainty with a not-so-dainty, bitter taste. They definitely can liven up a salad and almost any vegetable dish and are best enjoyed as a garnish or mixed with other sprouts. The larger microgreens can replace mixed greens in a salad.

DR. MARK HYMAN: "I'VE ALWAYS LOVED USING SPROUTS IN MY FOOD"

Mark Hyman, M.D., is a practicing family physician; ten-time number-one *New York Times* bestselling author; and internationally recognized leader, speaker, and educator. He is the director of the Cleveland Clinic Center for Functional Medicine and a regular medical contributor on several television programs. He is dedicated to tackling the root causes of chronic disease by harnessing the power of functional medicine to transform health care.

When were you first exposed to sprouts?
I've always loved using sprouts in my food. In college, I lived in a dorm where most folks were vegetarian and they liked to make big, beautiful salads using sprouts. I was fortunate to be surrounded by health-minded folks who prioritized real food from an early age.

What role do sprouts play in your work with functional medicine?

The most powerful tool you have to change your brain and your health is your fork. Food is not just calories or energy. Food contains information that talks to your genes, turning them on or off and affecting their function moment to moment. Food is the fastest-acting and most powerful medicine you can take to change your life. We call this nutrigenomics. *Think of your genes as the software that runs everything in your body. Just like your computer software, your genes only do what you instruct them to do with the stroke of your keyboard. The foods you eat are the keystrokes that send messages to your genes telling them what to do—creating health or disease. Among my favorite disease-fighting and health-promoting foods are plant foods such as sprouts, which are so nutrient dense that they provide your body with the best medicine. I tell my patients to include sprouts in their meals because they are a great source of nutrients like vitamin C, vitamin K, and fiber, which are really important for overall health.*

Since sprouts have so much more nutrition than their mature counterparts, why aren't they included in more dietary plans?

I don't think people know how nutritious sprouts are. It's up to us to spread the knowledge about these little powerhouses!

Can eating sprouts help us achieve our health goals?

Yes! Anytime you prioritize plant foods such as sprouts, you are preventing and helping to treat disease. This way of eating has a broad range of benefits for our health and beneficially affects our entire physiology, reducing inflammation, boosting detoxification, balancing hormones, and providing powerful antioxidant protection—all things that fix the underlying causes of disease.

Legume and Bean Sprouts

Legume and bean sprouts are by far the easiest sprouts to get started with. They can grow in glass jars (pages 127–130), trays (pages 140–142), and hemp bags (pages 133–137). They are the fastest seeds to sprout and reward you with a solid crunch and mild flavor. I love to fill up a bowl with a variety of these sprouts and put them out as a snack instead of nuts or pretzels. At first, people don't know what to think, but once they get started, they really get it, and the sprouts are gone. I even had an old friend from elementary school try to convince me to package up crunchy sprouts and sell them!

Eating legumes may help with many health issues, including reducing cholesterol levels and hypertension and the risk of diabetes, fibrocystic breast disease, and prostate cancer. Because they are so proteinaceous and hearty, they can help moderate blood sugar levels, not just at the meal but for hours afterward. And when you consume your legumes sprouted, the benefits increase by leaps and bounds!

WHAT ABOUT LECTINS?

Lectins are naturally occurring proteins that exist in plants; they are the plant's defense system and can act as antinutrients. Some research shows they can challenge digestion, potentially contributing to leaky gut and inflammation among other health concerns. Foods that contain lectins include fruits, vegetables, legumes, and grains. *And* there is a massive amount of scientific evidence that supports eating fruits, vegetables, legumes, and grains as part of a whole-food, plant-based diet. According to the Mayo Clinic, there is no evidence to show that eliminating dietary lectins will cure any medical disorders or conditions. But lectins don't provide any nutritional value, and it's possible that lectins may affect how you feel. What to do?

Enter sprouting. Soaking and then sprouting legumes (and grains too) decreases the lectin content, and the longer you sprout, the more the lectins are deactivated. The lectins in legumes are in the testa (seed coat), and as the seed germinates, the coat is metabolized and the lectins are reduced. One exception is the kidney bean; sprouted kidney beans are still really high in lectins. Therefore, it's recommended that sprouted kidney beans be cooked for at least ten minutes before eating them. Because this book focuses on sprouts that can be consumed raw, kidney beans aren't included in this chapter.

Adzuki Bean Sprouts

Adzuki beans have been harvested in Japan since 4000 B.C. They have been used as an ingredient in both savory and sweet foods as well as for medicinal purposes. Adzuki beans are one of my favorites and one of the easiest to sprout. They are crunchy, chewy, tasty, and filling, making them one of the best sprouts to snack on.

Where most beans are considered savory, adzukis are sweet without being high in sugars, making them perfect for diabetics and people who have a sweet tooth. Adzukis have a unique blend of protein, carbohydrates, and fiber that helps manage blood sugar levels. A 3½-ounce serving has almost twenty grams of protein and less than a gram of fat. That protein helps build muscle mass and lower body fat percentage. Their generous fiber is good for so many things, from weight loss to reversing coronary heart disease. The potassium and magnesium they contain work with the fiber to help regulate cholesterol, while the potassium relaxes blood vessels and increases blood flow. All of this is great for the heart! Try sprouted adzukis in a live-foods take on rice and beans (page 212).

Chickpea Sprouts

Chickpeas, also known as *garbanzo beans,* originated in the Middle East and have made their way around the world. They are currently the most widely consumed legume. Although tan chickpeas are the most recognizable variety, they come in other colors, including yellow, red, black, brown, and green. The nutritional properties of each colored variety are very similar, but the antioxidants change with the colors.

Chickpeas are popular for so many reasons. They taste great, and they are an excellent balance of protein, carbohydrates, and fiber with low amounts of fat. A single serving of chickpeas contains ten grams of protein (20 percent of the RDI) with only four grams of fat, mostly polyunsaturated. The protein-to-fat ratio is perfect for building muscle mass and losing extra weight. Compare that to a serving of steak, which has the same ten grams of protein but about eight grams of fat, mostly saturated. The steak will have zero dietary fiber, and the chickpeas will have a whopping seventeen grams (which is 68 percent of the RDI).

You can add chickpea sprouts to a salad, toss them with

chutneys to make the Indian street food chaat (page 189), or snack on them out of hand. You can even make hummus with them (pages 183–184). If everyone knew how delicious and nutritious sprouted hummus can be, we might start to see a shortage of raw chickpeas!

Green Pea Sprouts

The green pea, a.k.a. *pea* or *garden pea,* is an herbaceous annual plant that is grown around the world for its edible seeds. The wild plant is native in the Mediterranean region and has been traced all the way back to the Neolithic period.

Peas are a whole plant and are incredibly rich in so many vitamins and minerals. For example, peas are rich in niacin (vitamin B_3), with one cup containing almost 20 percent of the RDI. As is true for all the B vitamins, vitamin B_3 helps convert food into energy. Niacin is proven to lower "bad" (LDL) cholesterol by 5–20 percent. Not only that, but niacin also raises "good" (HDL) cholesterol by 15–35 percent. Count on sprouting those peas to exponentially increase their nutrient levels.

To someone who works out, the highlight of peas is protein. A single cup of sprouted peas contains more than 21 percent of the RDA for protein. That's 10.6 grams. Almost every Cross-Fit paleo gym enthusiast I've met has been blown away about swapping sprouted green peas for processed protein powders in their smoothies. Try the recipe on page 170 to upgrade your smoothie to 100 percent real food. Or try sprouted peas in a refreshing take on gazpacho (pages 179–180) or as the secret ingredient in avocado cream (page 217). Their flavor is slightly sweet and grassy.

Note that pea sprouts are different from pea shoots; turn to page 93 for more on them.

Lentil Sprouts

Lentils are a clear example of the magic of sprouting. They are fast—ready to eat in two to three days—and fairly foolproof. They are hearty, crunchy, and satisfying. They taste neutral to fantastic, which means that you can eat them alone or with many other foods and at any meal. They are divine in lentil mushroom pâté (pages 186–187), salads (page 210), and even smoothies (page 171).

Dry lentils have the second-highest antioxidant content of all tested legumes. Sprouted lentils have twice the antioxidant content as unsprouted, and red lentils beat other types in overall nutritive benefits. Lentils have an abundance of protein, iron, zinc, and folate. They are high in phytates, which may reduce the risk of colon cancer and may have protective effects against osteoporosis. Lentils may improve glycemic control even hours later or the next day (known as the "lentil effect") and therefore are great for people with diabetes and those looking to lose weight. Lentils contain the antinutrient phytic acid, but when they are sprouted, the phytic acid gets neutralized and more vitamins and minerals get absorbed.

Another fascinating aspect of sprouting lentils is what happens to the vitamin C. It literally increases over 400 percent from 5 percent to 21 percent of the RDA. Vitamin C is a well-known antioxidant that can help create collagen and reduce the signs of aging and the risk of cancer. There is no vitamin C in steak or chicken breast.

DR. MICHAEL GREGER: "A WHOLE FOOD PLUS"

Michael Greger, M.D., FACLM, is an internationally recognized lecturer, physician, and the founder of NutritionFacts .org, a public service that shares the latest in science and nutrition on your favorite foods to help you make the healthiest choices. He is the author of the *New York Times* bestseller *How Not to Die* and sprouts as often as he can.

How often do you eat sprouts?
I eat sprouts as frequently as I can when I'm not traveling. When I'm home, I always have jars going. Sometimes I'll have five jars set up at once so they are available daily.

Which are your favorite sprouts?
Broccoli and lentil sprouts are my go-tos. Broccoli for the sulforaphane and lentils for general nutrition. I also favor mung bean sprouts and adzuki sprouts.

What's the best thing about broccoli sprouts?
DIY broccoli sprouts have the biggest bang for the buck. A few years back, my calculations gave red cabbage the number-one spot, but it has since been one-upped by broccoli sprouts. Growing your own broccoli sprouts is one of the most cost-effective ways to improve your diet, and there certainly is enough research on broccoli sprouts to compel everyone on the planet to eat them.

How would you compare broccoli sprout supplements to eating fresh broccoli sprouts?

Using current technology, there is no comparison. So far, broccoli sprout supplements fall flat on their face.

With all the research on sprouts, why do you think they aren't much more widely eaten?

Sprouts are hard to sell on a wide scale because they are so perishable. Because they are hard to commercialize, there's little profit margin. Companies don't sell what's healthy; they sell what's profitable.

Can you eat too many sprouts?

Because lentil sprouts contain lectins, it is possible to eat too many. Soaking and sprouting lentils reduces the lectins—so much so that you eat a cup of lentil sprouts and all you have are benefits. But if you overdid it, you could get stomach cramps. That said, there's no reason everyone in the world shouldn't be eating lentil sprouts and broccoli sprouts every day.

What would be the difference between adding pea sprouts and a pea protein supplement to a smoothie?

One would be a whole food with infinitely more nutrition, and one would be a processed food that may have heavy metal contamination.

Do you consider sprouts to be a whole food?

They are a whole food plus! When you look at the nutrient density of sprouts, how can you beat them? All the nutrition is concentrated in a very small package. You add nothing but water, and all of a sudden you've made a plant with every single nutrient already there.

LENTIL SPROUTS VS. STEAK

Sprouted lentils have only 82 calories, 0 milligrams of cholesterol, and 10.4 grams of fat per 8-ounce serving. Compare that to steak, which has 614 calories, 177 milligrams of cholesterol, and 43 grams of fat—or even chicken breast, with 374 calories, 193 milligrams of cholesterol, and 8.1 grams of fat. You make the choice.

Mung Bean Sprouts

Carbonized mung beans have been discovered in archeological sites in India as far back as 4,500 years ago, and mung beans are currently widely grown in Asia, South America, Australia, and the United States. For reasons I have yet to understand, virtually all mung bean production is in Oklahoma. That being said, up to 75 percent of the mung beans consumed in the United States are imported.

The plant itself can grow one to five feet in length. They are self-pollinators and epigeal (meaning they grow close to the ground, not in the ground), making them very suitable for indoor sprouting. The seeds vary in size, shape, weight, and color with up to twelve thousand seeds per pound.

Sprouting is the preferred use for mung beans. Practically speaking, this makes sense, as one gram of seed will yield nine to ten grams of mung bean sprouts. Although I always recommend using organic seeds as your first choice, mung bean seeds generally are not treated with fungicides, insecticides, or bactericides because mung bean seeds are predominantly sold for sprouting purposes.

Mung beans are a powerhouse of vitamins and minerals. Vitamin C is a potent antioxidant that neutralizes free radicals, preventing them from attaching to healthy cells. We all need vitamin C, so you'll be happy to learn that the vitamin C content in mung beans goes from 1 percent to 23 percent when sprouted. Mung bean sprouts also contain hearty amounts of iron, folate, fiber, and manganese. A single cup has 43 percent of the RDI of vitamin K, which regulates bone mineralization and bone density and is essential for blood clotting.

Mung bean sprouts are hearty and can be added to almost any meal. They have a clean, nutty flavor that pairs well with fruits and vegetables. Because they have a high liquid content, you can use them in place of water in blending smoothies (page 170), raw soups (pages 179 to 182), and dips (pages 183–184). Or try them in an electrolyte drink (page 175) that contains two cups of mung bean sprouts in each serving!

There are two common types of mung bean sprouts: the mature ones that look like a two-inch white worm and the ones that look like the original mung bean with a little tail. They have similar nutrition and can come from the same seed. The difference is in how long they take to grow and how they taste. The two-inch sprouts are watery and crisp, and the smaller sprouts are more like a crunchy nut, similar to other legume sprouts.

SPROUTING CUTS CARBS

Sprouted mung beans provide fewer carbs than cooked, which will appeal to people on a high-protein, reduced-carb diet. While one cup of sprouted mung beans contains just six grams of carbs, a half cup of cooked mung beans gives you more than three times that amount. This is another stellar example of the many incredible benefits of sprouting.

Soybean Sprouts

During World War II, Dr. Clive M. McKay, professor of nutrition at Cornell University, wrote an article with this leading announcement: "Wanted! A vegetable that will grow in any climate, will rival meat in nutritive value, will mature in 3 to 5 days, may be planted any day of the year, will require neither soil nor sunshine, will rival tomatoes in vitamin C, will be free of waste in preparation and can be cooked with little fuel and as quickly as a . . . chop."

The suspect in question was soybean sprouts. McKay and his team of nutritionists had found that soybean sprouts show on average an increase of 300 percent in vitamin A and a 500–600 percent increase in vitamin C. Furthermore, in sprouting, starches are converted to simple sugars and are more easily digested. Thus sparked an interest in sprouts in the United States, decades before the hippies "discovered" this wonder food.

Like many other beans, soybeans originated in Southeast Asia, and Chinese farmers started domesticating them in approximately 1100 B.C. Within a few hundred years, they ended up in Japan and many other countries. Benjamin Franklin started growing soybeans in his garden before the Declaration of Independence. It took almost another hundred years before soybeans were grown by farmers in Illinois, Indiana, Iowa, Missouri, Nebraska, and Kansas. Today, soybeans are the dominant crops along with corn in the Corn Belt states. In the 1990s, the soybean had been genetically modified to withstand pesticides and herbicides so they could kill weeds without killing the soybean plant. Today, most soy in the United States is genetically modified.

There is a lot of controversy around soy products these days, and to cut to the chase, my recommendation is that if you want to include soy in your diet, only eat it in the following two ways: fermented in the form of tempeh, miso, or soy sauce; or sprouted.

One cup of soybean sprouts contain 9 percent of the RDI for protein, 15 percent of the RDI for folate, and 9 percent of the RDI for vitamin C. There is a known inverse correlation between soybean consumption and prostate and breast cancers. Researchers credit the substances daidzein and genistein that are found in soybeans. It is paramount to purchase organic soybean seeds to guarantee that they are not genetically modified. They can be swapped for mung bean sprouts; they are so similar most people would never notice.

STACY KENNEDY: "ADD SPROUTS TO WHAT YOU'RE ALREADY EATING"

Stacy Kennedy, M.P.H., R.D., C.S.O., L.D.N., is a board-certified specialist in oncology nutrition and senior clinical nutritionist for Dana-Farber / Brigham and Women's Cancer Center, Harvard Medical School teaching affiliates, in Boston. She teaches nutrition at Simmons College and cofounded her private practice, Wellness Guides LLC.

As a dietician, what do you like best about sprouts?
They're a food—not a pill—so you get to eat them! Eating sprouts is an effective way of delivering a high amount of nutrients in a compact food source. Sprouts go well with a lot of foods we're already eating. That means we all can wrap our heads around them, which is great, because from a nutritional standpoint, there are so many benefits to including sprouts in our diet.

What are some of those benefits?
Because sprouts are nutrient dense, they give us the most bang for our buck. As busy people, so many of us are looking for simple things to provide us with true nutrition. Nutrient-wise, you can pick out some heroes like protein and fiber, but what I really like about sprouts is that they are a food you can eat on a recurring basis easily and conveniently. And there is potential benefit for the microbiome; as that field continues to grow, we will learn more about the role sprouts can play.

What's the best way of getting sprouts into people's diets?
I find one of the biggest challenges in working with my patients is radically shifting their eating styles. This is rarely effective, and at the end of the day, to consistently include certain foods and to want to be able to do so is what is really going to help the most. This is why I'd advocate adding sprouts to what you're already eating, such as sandwiches or salads, at least when you're starting out.

They fit nicely into just about any diet your doctor or nutritionist might have you on.

Who should eat sprouts?
Sprouts are a basic food that's accessible for everyone. Just about anyone, from my students in their early twenties to my mom, can wrap their heads around them, and they all should eat them!

SHOOTS

Shoots are an important part of any sprouting kitchen. They provide a diversity of flavors, textures, and nutrition, and growing them will keep you on the ball. Shoots are the greenest and heartiest seed sprout, making them perfect as a lettuce replacement for salad. I prefer eating a blend of sunflower shoots and pea shoots over any mature leafy green. These specialty crops can be grown indoors very fast. The seed itself provides all the nutrients to get them to edible size, about two inches. If they are sprouted in soil, you can let them grow all the way to six inches by continuing to spray them with water and providing them with access to normal daylight (not direct sunlight). They turn into small plants that get harvested at the base of the stem and are eaten whole. They are heliotropic, meaning they grow toward the light. They grow quickly and vertically and therefore do best in soil or a sprouting medium, which could be as simple as a couple of sheets of unbleached paper towels. They get soaked overnight and then transferred to the sprouting medium. See pages 153–156 for detailed instructions for growing shoots.

Pea Shoots

Pea shoots, the young plant of a pea, are a crowd favorite because they are sweet and tender with crispy, chewy stems. The flavor is similar to field peas, but milder. If you're looking to incorporate wheatgrass juice into your routine (see pages 144–146) but find it a little too intense, try making a blended juice of 50 percent pea shoots at first and work your way up to all wheatgrass (or continue with the blend if you are happy there). Pea shoots are naturally low in calories and are a great source of beta-carotene, vitamin C, folate, and both soluble and insoluble fiber. They are a wonderful replacement for or adjunct to baby greens in salads and go very well with sunflower sprouts. Try tucking a handful into a wrap instead of lettuce.

Unlike the pea sprout (see pages 83–84), which is mostly pea with a small sprout shooting forth and which is eaten whole, pea shoots are grown in soil or a sprouting medium. They generally grow two to six inches tall and have edible leaves and immature tendrils on them. One of the reasons for their popularity is that they have the flavor of the pea but can be grown indoors in a fraction of the time. They taste like springtime, but you get to eat them all year round!

Sunflower Shoots

Sunflower seeds are extremely versatile and can be sprouted and consumed in a variety of ways. These are the top ones in my playbook:

1. Whole sunflower seeds used to grow sunflower shoots
2. Hulled sunflower seeds that are sprouted in a jar and eaten like a legume sprout
3. Hulled sunflower seeds that are soaked overnight to begin the germination process and then dried in a dehydrator or low-temperature oven and eaten like a traditional nut or seed

Sunflower sprouts, which actually are shoots en route to becoming a microgreen, are one of the most loved and revered sprouts. Even un-health nuts who shun sprouts actually like the texture and taste of sunflower sprouts. The small leaves have a deep texture with a flavor reminiscent of a sweet almond. They are not spicy and have a satisfying chew, which makes them a great part of a salad or a salad all to itself.

Only a small amount of fresh sunflower sprouts contains more than one hundred enzymes. And sunflower sprouts contain a high amount of zinc, which is responsible for numerous functions in the body, including activating T lymphocytes (T cells), which regulate immune responses and attack infected or cancerous cells. They are high in B vitamins and folic acid, which helps develop a growing fetus's nervous system, and they can help prevent clogging of a mother's milk ducts while breast-feeding. For men, they not only promote healthy sperm, they have been linked to decreased risk of age-related chronic disease and macular degeneration.

Sunflower sprouts are dry and hearty and travel well for several hours. They can be eaten as a snack or added to almost any dish. They are one of the bestselling sprouts and can easily be grown at home in a tray with or without soil (see pages 140–143).

Grasses

Wheatgrass and barley grass have been part of the health food phenomenon for the last forty or so years, for good reason. Other than their intense taste, there are seemingly only upsides to consuming the juice that is made from them. Other grasses, such as barley grass, oat grass, spelt grass, and rye grass, are similar and can be sprouted, grown, and used interchangeably. They all taste like grass, but as you become a connoisseur, you will start to distinguish the subtle differences and choose your favorites.

Although it has the word *wheat* in the name, the blades of grass that are consumed do not contain any gluten. The grass does come from the wheat berry, so if you are highly sensitive to wheat or gluten or have celiac disease, it may be best to avoid it so as not to introduce wheat into your kitchen. The same precautions go for spelt, barley, and rye, as all three contain gluten. When in doubt, check with a health-care provider.

All forms of wheatgrass, ranging from fresh to frozen juice to tablets and powders, include chlorophyll, flavonoids, vitamins C and E, and host of antioxidants. There is extensive research being performed on the medical use of wheatgrass. Several studies indicate that wheatgrass may help lower cholesterol levels, kill cancer cells, aid in blood sugar regulation, reduce inflammation, and help with weight loss. See pages 144–146 to learn how to sprout wheatgrass and other grasses for juicing.

HOW WHEATGRASS SAVED ME FROM SURGERY

By the time I was thirty-three, I was so fed up with not being able to breathe through my nose that I finally went to the Manhattan Eye, Ear, and Throat Hospital to see a specialist. My intention was to get surgery to "fix" my deviated septum. After waiting six weeks for the appointment and another two hours in the waiting room, the surgeon came in to speak with me. He was handsome, well spoken, and well put together, and I felt like I was on a movie set. He made me feel very comfortable until he said something that really triggered me. I thought he was joking, but much to my surprise, he was serious, serious as a heart attack. He started to show me pictures and asked me what I wanted my nose to look like. I said that I wasn't there for plastic surgery, I was there because I couldn't breathe through my nose. He said that he knew that, but since we were up there, we might as well kill two birds with one stone. I resisted the temptation to give him a piece of my mind (this was before I became a meditator) and decided to just leave. That probably was one of the best decisions of my life.

I told one of my friends what happened at the hospital, and he responded that it sounded like mucus caused by what I was eating and that I probably could fix it without surgery. He recommended that I see the alternative doctor he was going to for back pain. I eagerly arranged an appointment and went to see him. It was a very different setup from the hospital on the Upper East Side. It was a small space on the fourteenth floor of an office building. I opened the door to see about six people sitting, standing, bending, or pressing against the wall doing his custom stretching exercises. A young woman came out from behind a closed door, which turned out to be the examining room. She asked my name and had me fill out paperwork. I sat patiently on the floor until it was my turn to see the doctor, who was legally blind. He took my nose between his fingers and bent it toward my left ear and then toward my right ear, and then he pushed it up and down. He proceeded to tell me that there was nothing physically wrong with my nose or my septum. The problem was my diet—it was mucus forming, inflammatory—and that I wasn't breathing properly. He told me to give up all dairy and that I should start consuming copious amounts of wheatgrass juice. So wheatgrass juice shots became part of my daily routine.

A few weeks later, I was struggling to overcome seasonal sickness, a mild case of the common cold, and rather than turn to over-the-counter medications from the pharmacy, I sought out wheatgrass juice. I raced to the closest health food store, on Sixth Avenue and Ninth Street in the West Village. I arrived at the store fifteen minutes before they closed and was ecstatic to have made it in the nick of time. But when I asked for a shot of wheatgrass, the juice bar attendant informed me they had already cleaned the wheatgrass juicer. For anyone familiar with juicing, this can be a tedious and lengthy process. I couldn't convince them to serve me, so seeing a flat of wheatgrass growing on the counter, I grabbed a handful, uprooted the small blades of green goodness, and stuffed them into my mouth. Chewing slowly, I savored each and every bit of juice extracted from the blades of grass and then spit out the cellulose and fiber. The wheatgrass juice had an immediate impact on my emotional and physical state. All of a sudden, I had more energy and felt alive. I began a conversation and forgot that I wasn't feeling well just a few minutes prior.

You may have noticed flats of wheatgrass at your farmers' market or grocery store; you can also grow wheatgrass in your own home; turn to pages 144–146 to learn how.

STEPHEN FISKELL: THIRTY DAYS OF SPROUTS

Stephen Fiskell lives in San Francisco, where he recently left his job in technology to pursue a path of personal health. I met Stephen under a waterfall in Bali, where we talked about veganism, and he set an intention to go on a thirty-day sprout cleanse. I spoke to him about his super-sprout experience.

What inspired you to go on a thirty-day sprout cleanse?
It was time for a hard reset. I had been overweight all my life, and I was looking to build a new relationship with food. One impetus to lose the weight was to get in shape for ultra-running, a passion of mine.

What did your meals look like?
I was eating all things sprouts and nothing else, except for the occasional dash of hot sauce to spice them up. I'd go to the supermarket and get containers of clover, broccoli, sunflower, and mixed bean sprouts. I was eating up to fifteen different types of sprouts. I hadn't even known there were that many sprouts to begin with! I experimented with cooking the sprouts a few times, but since sprouts are mostly water, the whole container would turn into a single bite of food, and it wasn't tasty.

Did you grow your own sprouts?
I'd go to the supermarket and buy all *the sprouts. I realized I needed more protein, and that was when I started growing my own bean sprouts to supplement what I would find at the store. Sprouting at home has helped me to connect to the food I eat.*

What did your friends think?

My roommates were curious and supportive. It was a mixed reaction at work. My buddy who got me into veganism did a day of solidarity with me by eating only mung bean sprouts for the entire day.

How did you feel during the thirty days?

Great! I always ate until I was full and didn't need more food. My cravings went away, and I ran a twelve-hour ultramarathon fueled by sprouts. The five days prior to the marathon, I ate about five hundred calories in sprouts a day (which is a lot of sprouts!), and I brought one thousand calories' worth of sprouts to the race. I completed the ultramarathon, and the next day, I was a little sore, and the day after that, I was completely fine. It was mind-blowing! Over the course of the month, I lost twenty-four pounds. My take-away was that you don't need as much food as you think; in the end, it's the quality of the food that matters.

GRAINS, NUTS, AND SEEDS

Grains

All seeds must be sprouted to become mature plants. Grains are no exception, and as a matter of fact, many whole grains are sprouted on a very regular basis. Among the popular grains are alfalfa, amaranth, clover, corn, quinoa, wheat, barley, rye, spelt, millet, rice, and oats.

Whole grains contain the germ, the endosperm, the outer bran layer, and sometimes a hard testa. The germ contains the embryo with all the oils and nutrients required to activate the seed into a blossoming plant. There is no one playbook for all grains. Alfalfa is sprouted like a salad green, and some rice won't sprout because it has been overly processed after harvesting, but many grains sprout easily and provide enormous nutrition.

Because grains sprout so fast, they aren't readily commercially available. That's actually good for you. By controlling the process, you get to ensure that they are safe and fresh. Not to mention the money you will save by sprouting at home.

Grains are considered a health food, and sprouted grains are considered a superfood. Research from Cornell University going back to the 1940s demonstrated that sprouting can increase vitamin A by 300 percent and vitamin C by 500 percent. There is research indicating that sprouted brown rice fights diabetes and cardiovascular disease and even decreases depression and fatigue in nursing mothers. Among the nutrients sprouted grains contain are folate, iron, vitamin C, zinc, magnesium, and protein. Germination breaks down a percentage of the starchy endosperm and removes antinutrients, making them easier to digest than unsprouted grains. So if you've been thinking of giving up grains, first try sprouting them!

Sprouted grains are a good complement to sprouted veggies for taste, texture, variety, and flavor. Try sprouted quinoa tabbouleh (pages 202–203), buckwheat cereal (pages 177–178), or oatmeal. Once you go sprouted, you can't go back.

Nuts and Edible Seeds

I've always enjoyed eating nuts and seeds, especially peanuts (even though I know now that they are a legume), walnuts, almonds, cashews, Brazil nuts, macadamia nuts, hazelnuts, hemp seeds, sunflower seeds, and pumpkin seeds. The problem for me was that I was eating them in roasted and salted form, which made them hard to stop eating and also hard to digest. I have since been schooled on the fact that added fats and salts make you want to eat more of them.

Then I began eating nuts and seeds raw, and that was a significant improvement. I would stop eating them after I was no longer hungry. I didn't have to go all the way to full. Finally, I discovered soaking and sprouting nuts and seeds before eating them to remove the enzyme inhibitors and activate them. The soaking would be for as little as eight to twenty-four hours with a few rinses along the way. Then I would let them sun-dry for a day—one of the benefits of living in the Mojave Desert. (If you don't have access to full-on sun, you can use a dehydrator or your oven on the lowest setting. Ideally, you want to dry them slowly at temperatures below 116°F to get them ready for snacking.)

Soaking and sprouting nuts and seeds became a whole new ball game. Now I could eat them, enjoy them, *and* digest them. Several recipes in the book call for sprouted nuts and seeds as an adjunct to your veggie-sprouting routine. These include sprouted almond milk (page 169), sprouted tahini (page 216), halvah (pages 228–229), and a raw sprouted brownie (pages 226–227).

Almonds, cashews, macadamia nuts, Brazil nuts, hazelnuts, pumpkin seeds, pecans, hulled sunflower, and hemp seeds all benefit from soaking before adding to recipes. With the exception of sunflower seeds and almonds if you are lucky, nuts and seeds will sprout. They will get bigger and then shrink a bit as they dry.

Sprouting Chart

SEED	SPROUTING METHODS	SEED QUANTITY	SOAK AND RINSE TIME	SPROUTING AND SPRAYING TIME	MICROGREEN SPRAYING TIME	YIELD SPROUTS	YIELD MICROGREENS
SALAD SPROUTS							
Alfalfa	jar, bag, tray	¼ cup	8 hours	3–5 days		4 cups	
Basil (best as a microgreen)	jar, bag, tray	¼ cup	8 hours		7–14 days		6 cups
Broccoli	jar, bag, tray	¼ cup	8 hours	3–5 days		4 cups	
Cabbage	jar, bag, tray	¼ cup	8 hours	3–5 days		4 cups	
Celery (best as a microgreen)	jar, bag, tray	¼ cup	8 hours		12–20 days		2 cups
Clover	jar, bag, tray	¼ cup	8 hours	3–5 days		4 cups	
Fenugreek	jar, bag, tray	¼ cup	8 hours	3–5 days		4 cups	
Hemp (unhulled)	jar, bag, tray	¼ cup	8 hours	3–5 days		4 cups	
Onion	jar, bag, tray	¼ cup	8 hours	3–5 days		4 cups	
Radish	jar, bag, tray	¼ cup	8 hours	3–5 days		4 cups	
Watercress	jar, bag, tray	¼ cup	8 hours	3–5 days		4 cups	

SEED	SPROUTING METHODS	SEED QUANTITY	SOAK AND RINSE TIME	SPROUTING AND SPRAYING TIME	MICROGREEN SPRAYING TIME	YIELD SPROUTS	YIELD MICROGREENS
GELATINOUS SPROUTS							
Arugula	clay, tray	¼ cup	spray immediately	5–7 days		4 cups	
Chia	clay, tray	¼ cup	spray immediately	5–7 days		4 cups	
Flax	clay, tray	¼ cup	spray immediately	5–7 days		4 cups	
Mustard (slightly gelatinous)	clay, tray	¼ cup	spray immediately	5–7 days		4 cups	
LEGUME AND BEAN SPROUTS							
Adzuki bean	jar, bag	½ cup	8 hours	2–3 days		1 cup	
Chickpea	jar, bag	½ cup	8 hours	2–3 days		1 cup	
Green pea	jar, bag	½ cup	8 hours	2–3 days		1 cup	
Lentil	jar, bag	½ cup	8 hours	2–3 days		1 cup	
Mung bean (young)	jar, bag	½ cup	8 hours	2–3 days		1 cup	
Mung bean (mature)	jar, bag	½ cup	8 hours	7–10 days		4 cups	
Soybean	jar, bag	½ cup	8 hours	2–3 days		1 cup	

SEED	SPROUTING METHODS	SEED QUANTITY	SOAK AND RINSE TIME	SPROUTING AND SPRAYING TIME	MICROGREEN SPRAYING TIME	YIELD SPROUTS	YIELD MICRO-GREENS
SHOOTS							
Pea	tray, bag	½ cup	8 hours	7–10 days	10–15 days		1¼ cups
Sunflower	tray, bag	½ cup	8 hours	7–10 days	10–15 days		1¼ cups
Buckwheat	tray	½ cup	8 hours	7–10 days	10–15 days		1¼ cups
WHEATGRASS AND OTHER GRASSES							
Wheatgrass	tray	2 cups	12 hours	7–10 days	10–15 days		1¼ cups
Barley grass	tray	2 cups	12 hours	7–10 days	10–15 days		1¼ cups
Oat grass	tray	2 cups	12 hours	7–10 days	10–15 days		1¼ cups
GRAINS							
Buckwheat (unhulled)	tray	½ cup	30 minutes	5–7 days	10–15 days		4 cups
Oats	jar	½ cup	12 hours	2–3 days		1½ cups	
Quinoa	jar, bag	½ cup	4 hours	1–2 days		1 cup	

SEED	SPROUTING METHODS	SEED QUANTITY	SOAK AND RINSE TIME	SPROUTNG AND SPRAYING TIME	MICROGREEN SPRAYING TIME	YIELD SPROUTS	YIELD MICROGREENS
NUTS AND EDIBLE SEEDS							
Almonds	jar, bag	½ cup	8 hours	1–2 days		¾ cup	
Sesame seeds (unhulled)	jar, bag	½ cup	4 hours	1–2 days		¾ cup	
Sesame seeds (hulled)	jar, bag	½ cup	4 hours	1–2 days		¾ cup	
Sundflower seeds (hulled)	jar, bag	½ cup	4 hours	1–2 days		¾ cup	
Hemp (hulled)	jar, bag	½ cup	4 hours	1–2 days		¾ cup	
Pumpkin (hulled)	jar, bag	½ cup	4 hours	1–2 days		¾ cup	

YOUR SPROUT GARDEN

A Radically Simple Setup

to Eat Locally in Any Season

on Any Budget

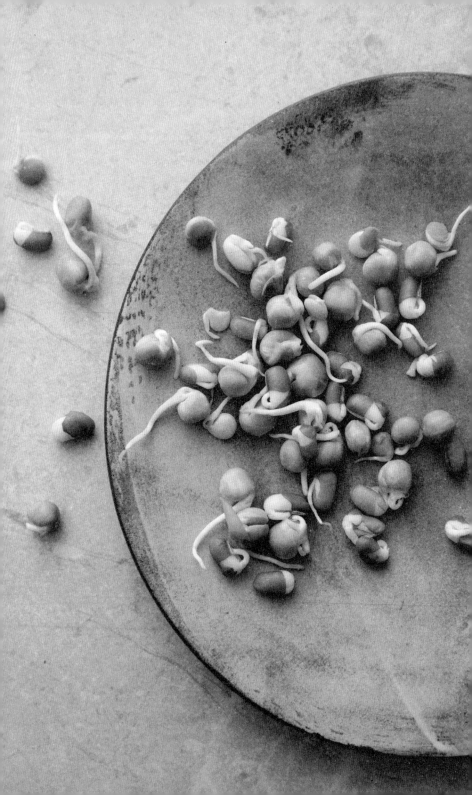

I POUR MY heart out about sprouts to anyone who will listen—friends, neighbors, random people on the street, you, the reader. If I've succeeded in getting their attention, the first question they'll ask inevitably is "How can I get started?" My answer is that it can be as easy as a trip to a grocery store or as adventurous as creating your own personal sprout garden.

Not everybody has a green thumb. But *everybody* has a sprouting hand. Sprouting couldn't be easier. You start with shelf-stable seeds, soak them in water for a few hours, drain, rinse periodically, and wait a few days until the magical transformation of seed to sprout occurs. Sprouts are just dying to come alive and reach their full potential!

Anyone and everyone can grow sprouts, and growing your own is the best way of ensuring your sprouts are the freshest and tastiest possible. Sprouting at home saves you money and means you are in control of the process and the type and amount of produce you get to enjoy. (But if you don't have the time, space, or inclination to sprout, buying sprouts at the store is a completely doable option, and all the recipes in the book can be made with store-bought sprouts. See page 126 for tips on safely using sprouts from the store.)

This chapter is my rogue, relentless, creative, and resourceful approach to sprouting. My goal is for you to eat sprouts because, as you have learned in the Sprout Primer (pages 55 to 105), sprouts are off the charts on almost every single health front.

Choose Your Seed

The seed is a dormant plant that will come to life with just a little water, a process called *germination*. Once the seed is germinated, typically by soaking for several hours, we can determine the path for it. Some seeds can sprout in as little as eight hours, and some require as much as eight weeks. In this time, the seed changes its metabolic state from a dry, hard, pebble-like structure to a life force that can help feed the planet.

I have dreams of the future of sprouting. An inexpensive machine that can automate the entire sprouting process. This isn't a pure fantasy because it actually can be done. In my lab, we have assembled most of the technology that is required to make this happen. But the good thing for you, the reader, farmer, saint, and lover, is that you don't need anything that fancy. You can do it all on your own with the simplest of tools and determination.

All you need to get started is seeds. The universe for seeds is quite vast, and almost all seeds can be made into food. With your seeds and a vessel to sprout them in, you are ready to sprout. There are various sprouters on the market, which I'll cover in the following pages, but for starters, your simplest and cheapest options are a mason jar with a mesh screen, a dedicated sprouting bag, or even a sterilized window screen.

Seeds can be found sold in bags, boxes, bulk bins, and on the internet via mail order, and you'll increasingly find them in farmers' markets. The goal is to grow edible, nutritious sprouts, and to do so, I highly recommend that you purchase organic seeds that were grown specifically for sprouting. These types of seeds have very high germination rates, ensuring successful sprouting. Seeds tend to look more or less the same, but they don't all act the same. The sprouting industry has become a lot more sophisticated, and it's possible today to find vendors both online and off that sell seeds specifically designed for sprouting that are USDA certified organic, that have been tested for high germination rates, and have been prewashed to reduce or eliminate harmful bacteria. Let's learn the language of seeds by asking some questions.

Where are the seeds from?

This matters a lot, because it's possible that your seeds are organic, heirloom, and grown on a little farm ten miles away from you, or they could be contaminated by exposure to an environment polluted by bacteria, fungus, chemicals, or a nuclear power plant. This is a very real concern. Foodies find it fascinating to learn where their food comes from, with whole movements supporting products grown in place, from CSAs, to urban rooftop gardens, to the birth of "Made in Brooklyn." Where your food comes from also could have a direct impact on your health. What's the best way to truly know your source?

Get curious. The more you participate, the more conscious and present you will be when you eat, and the whole eating experience becomes way more interesting. Think of it like a baseball game. It's your home team, and you know every player, their stats, where they are from, and so on. You're really pumped! Then imagine going to a rugby game in another country where they speak another language. The whole cultural experience is fascinating and the adrenaline is palpable, but you know nothing about the game or the players, and you can't quite connect in the way you did with your home team. The takeaway: Read your labels! Many products will not only provide the source but a description of the source as well. The companies on pages 233–234 are my current go-tos, but keep in mind that sources are always changing as the world changes. If the label leaves you with lingering questions, don't be afraid to email or call the company.

Are they high-germination seeds?

Inside every seed is a plant that lies dormant until it's soaked and then ready for sprouting. Germination is that seed fulfilling its destiny: growing into a plant. You may think that every seed grows into a plant, but this is not always the case. Some seeds just don't make it, for a number of possible reasons:

1) They sat on the shelf too long.
2) They were irradiated.
3) They were chipped, cracked, broken into pieces, or otherwise damaged.
4) They were partially eaten or contaminated by pests.

5) They were exposed to water and developed mold.

6) They were genetically modified or hybridized for a specific outcome other than sprouting, such as nutrition or weight for resale. For example, you occasionally will find a small white or black seed in seedless watermelons; these seeds will be more likely *not* to sprout than to sprout.

7) They are not truly raw (a cooked seed will not sprout).

When I first got turned on to a plant-based lifestyle and started eating "raw," I chose chickpeas for protein and set out to sprout them to unleash their life force within. So I'd head over to the bulk bin, go home with a supply of organic chickpeas, and set them up for sprouting. It was hit or miss, and I wondered why until I learned that not all seeds are equal. I needed to look specifically for dedicated seeds for sprouting. Search for the term *high-germination* on the label, and if you're curious about germination rates, don't be afraid to question the company. I've seen germination rates range from 50–90 percent, so it pays to ask! The seeds recommended on pages 233–234 are all high-germination seeds.

Are the seeds organic?

There are pockets of the world where farming, gardening, and tending to the environment with loving care are a very high priority. (My friend and cowriter, Leda Scheintaub, tells me Brattleboro, Vermont, where she lives, is one of them. If you've never visited, perhaps you'll consider it. Brattleboro would be thrilled to have you!) But unfortunately, profit trumps everything else most of the time, and even seeds for sprouting—a commodity we might consider inherently health-supportive—could be coming from an unhealthy environment. Although there have been manic media stories against the case for organic, I have found that these arguments are flawed. Let's put aside the debate on whether organic is more nutritious than conventional and consider whether or not your produce is sprayed with poisonous chemicals and grown with synthetic fertilizers, something I believe no one would want to ingest given the choice. My point of view is very conservative: I opt for organic, preferably heirloom seeds that are as natural and traceable as possible.

But if you do not see the USDA certified organic label on your sprout seeds or sprouts, it's time to ask questions again! Becoming certified organic is a time-consuming, lengthy process, and tight profit margins mean some growers that do not spray their seeds opt not to certify. Instead, they develop trusted relationships with their customers and educate them on their sources. If your seeds are organic, by default they also are non-GMO. Genetic modification introduces new traits to plants that are not inherently there, such as resistance to pests or herbicides. My biggest gripe with genetically modified (GM) plants is that the pesticide levels on the food are too high. If the goal is to grow a lot, we certainly have met that goal: Between 1986 and 2016, we have seen a tenfold increase in the number of hectares of cropland. But at what cost? These pesticides, most famously Monsanto's Roundup, are absorbed into the plants and ultimately our bodies. The GM seeds are tolerant of the Roundup, but everything else gets extinguished. See the sidebar for more on this sorry state of seeds.

WHY ORGANIC MATTERS

When purchasing certified organic seed (and other foods), you are guaranteed that you are buying seeds that explicitly do not contain genetically modified organisms (GMOs) or genetically engineered (GE) seeds. Organic also guarantees that the farmer is not using synthetic chemicals, pesticides, herbicides, fungicides, or insecticides. By actually working the land, the farmer gets better soil and topsoil, conserves water, increases fertility, and reduces soil erosion. Organic farming is better for the air quality, ground quality, and water quality that affects all living animals, including human animals, and other creatures in the surrounding area.

The chemical spraying and cancer connection are becoming all too real. In a systematic review of cancer health effects from pesticides, six medical doctors across family practices, oncology departments, and universities reviewed eighty-three primary peer-reviewed studies and found that seventy-two had positive associations between pesticide use and specific types of cancer, including lung, breast, pancreatic, brain, prostate, stomach, and kidney and non-Hodgkin's lymphoma and leukemia. The study concluded that there is enough evidence to recommend that patients reduce the use of pesticides.

The case against pesticides, in particular Monsanto's Roundup, was brought to the public's eye when Dewayne Johnson filed suit against the corporation in 2018. Mr. Johnson developed what appeared to be a bad rash, but it was in fact symptoms of non-Hodgkin's lymphoma. His case was relatively simple: He argued that Monsanto's Roundup likely caused his disease. His lawyers also attested that Monsanto failed to warn consumers about the risks. After only three days of deliberation, Mr. Johnson was awarded $250 million in punitive damages and an additional $39 million in compensatory damages.

All that money, or in fact all the money in the world, will most likely not save him. "The jury found Monsanto acted with malice and oppression because they knew what they were doing was wrong and doing it with reckless disregard for human life," said Robert F. Kennedy Jr. Although Monsanto is denying any wrongdoing, this is just the first of hundreds of cancer-patient cases against Monsanto. The smoking gun was the confidential, secret internal documents proving that Monsanto has known for decades that Roundup could cause cancer.

It's no wonder then that in the United States (according to research from the Hartman Group), many consumers prefer organic because of the perception of fewer chemicals, higher quality, and food that is healthier for you and better for the world. As a matter of fact, the vast majority of U.S. consumers report using organic and/or natural food and beverage products, with about a third of them using them on at least a weekly basis.

I encourage you to go organic when you sprout. If you don't think you can afford it, see the math on pages 125–126 and think again.

Have the seeds been tested for pathogens, including *E. coli,* listeria, and salmonella?

How meticulous a grower's food quality and safety program is will give you peace of mind in the short term and longevity in the long term. According to the FDA, the seed is typically the source of the bacteria. There are a number of approved techniques to kill harmful bacteria that may be present on seeds and tests to ensure that the process was effective. If the label does not indicate that the seeds have been tested, pick up the phone and ask or send an email to customer service.

What is the shelf life of the seeds?

Seeds are alive, and although theoretically they can remain dormant for centuries, they also can be relatively perishable and over time become less vital, with their germination rate decreasing over time. It comes down to common sense: Like most food sold, it's important to abide by the use-by date of your seeds.

What is the ideal protocol to sprout the seeds in?

There are extensive instructions in this book about how to sprout your individual seeds, and it's also useful to get the instructions from the source. As there are infinite varieties and sources for seeds, there may be specific nuances or tips that will help you get the best results.

How much will my seeds yield?

To the newbie, sprouting can be a mystery. Dive in, and prepare to be astounded by their growth! Some seeds will merely double their size, and some will grow more than ten times. For example, ½ cup of mung beans will yield 2½ cups of sprouts in six to seven days, while ¼ cup of alfalfa seeds will yield 8 cups of alfalfa sprouts in just five to seven days. This certainly will affect your sprouting plans, in particular when you are making the recipes from this book. Refer to the sprouting growth chart on pages 102–105 for the ratio of seeds to final sprouts.

What is the nutritional content of the seeds?

If there were a competition for most nutrient-dense food, sprouts would win the gold medal. For starters, sprouts have twenty to thirty times the nutrients of other vegetables and one hundred times those of meat. Sprouting packs in vitamins, micronutrients, phytonutrients, minerals, flavonoids, polyphenols, antioxidants, prebiotics, probiotics, and live enzymes. The more you home in on the nutrition of the individual sprouts you are eating, the more excited, enthusiastic, and motivated you will be to eat those sprouts. Just like vegetables, different sprouts contain different types and amounts of nutrients. For example, mung bean sprouts are a great source for folate, magnesium, and protein; sulforaphane is found in broccoli sprouts; and chia seed sprouts are high in omega-3 fatty acids. See the Sprout Primer (pages 55 to 105) for stats on individual sprouts and their role in targeted nutrition.

Do my seeds need fertilizer?

The only case in which fertilizer would be helpful is if you are growing sprouts on a paper towel or non-soil-based growing medium, such as from coconut husk or hemp fibers. These are typically one-eighth to one-quarter inch thick, feel like felt, and hold water long enough between sprays to keep the seeds moist. Fertilizer will help your shoots grow longer and is especially useful if you eventually plan to plant your seeds in soil. My preferred fertilizer is a liquid seaweed called *kelp* (see Resources, pages 233–234). Dilute one teaspoon into one quart of water and fill up a dedicated spray bottle. Spray the seeds once or twice a day.

Add Water

To grow sprouts, all you really need are great seeds and the best water source you can find. Seeds are hungry for water so they can be activated. They are alive and waiting to get out of their state of dormancy to a state of germination.

You as a budding sprouting scientist can do a test of your tap water: Use the same amount of seeds and water, but switch up your water source and track the results. In some places in the world, tap water is fine. In many other cases, it may have too many contaminants. Polluted water can be like putting out a candle with a firehose and can act to deter or prevent your seeds from sprouting. Your seeds will tell you if they dig your water source.

MY JOURNEY OFF THE WATER GRID

I am passionate about water and think it's a shame that not every faucet in our country produces water good enough for sprouting. But with a little experimentation and a water filter, you should be able to fix whatever is wrong with your water.

For the past twenty years, my preferred drinking water has come from natural springs where I get the honor of harvesting the water myself. To be clear, I don't just go to any stream, puddle, or septic system and drink the water! The water must be flowing right out of the ground or mountain in such a way that it fills a bottle directly. I always go to a known source where people have been drinking that water for decades. In many cases, I will fund the testing of the water with a certified lab that specializes in drinking water. One of my favorite springs is called Red Rock, near Stinson Beach in Northern California. Locals in Mill Valley, Stinson Beach, San Francisco, Oakland, and even San José source the water from there. If you didn't know where it was, it would be easy to drive by and miss it, but the cars parked by the side of the road, with trunks open and people loading various size bottles of water, is a dead giveaway. This spring has been tested consistently for everything from mineral content to coliform bacteria. After severe rains and landslides, they closed that road and access to the spring, but the spring was still flowing. Countless people that I know made treks over the mountain, up the road, and down the road in the early morning or late at night to source the water. I will take the Fifth on whether one of those people was me.

Today, I live deep in the Mojave Desert, way off the traditional water grid. After decades in the raw vegan world and cold-pressed juice world, I wanted to get back to nature and away from the noise. I moved to a small plot of land in the valley of an old lake bed and put up a fifteen-foot-diameter Burning Man yurt. Not a lot grows here, and there are no hot and cold running water services provided by the town. As a matter of fact, my town isn't even incorporated, and in the 150-mile radius of the town, there are only about 650 people. The desert is pretty harsh, and only the strong and flexible survive. The weather in the Mojave can swing from 20 to 120 degrees in a six-month period. The blazing sun dries out everything in the summer, and the frost will freeze everything else. And there are just two options for water: dig a well (365+ feet) or have it hauled in with a water truck

like in the movie *Mad Max*. As it turns out, my well has a
TDS (total dissolved solids) number of around 1,600, where
the preferred level is 50–100. In order to drink my water, I
had to install a commercial four-stage reverse-osmosis water
filtration system that brings the water below that level, and
I remineralize it with fresh lemon wedges. Growing anything
here is a challenge, except sprouts and some fruit trees that
like brackish water. I can manage to sprout 365 days a year.
My sprouting systems are set up to use the least amount of
water for soaking and rinsing the seeds as possible, and then I
take the used water from the seeds to water the mature native
plants growing out on my land. This really makes me happy,
and the enormous yields I get from my sprouts are incredible.

Go Forth and Sprout Safely

According to the Centers for Disease Control and Prevention,
there are an estimated 9.4 million foodborne illnesses from
known pathogens annually. There are approximately 800 foodborne outbreaks annually in the United States with approximately 15,000 illnesses, 800 hospitalizations, and 20 deaths.
According to FoodSafety.gov, there have been at least 21 reported outbreaks associated with sprouts between 2009 and
2015. That's less than 4 per year out of the 5,760 outbreaks. For
comparison purposes, fish had 222 reported outbreaks, beef
had 106, dairy had 136, chicken had 123, pork had 89, and
turkey had 50. According to FoodSafety.gov, sprouts carry a
risk of illness like any fresh produce. Their advice is to reduce
the risk of illness; children, the elderly, and pregnant women
should avoid eating raw sprouts of any kind.

This perspective doesn't surprise me since there are no lobbying groups in Washington, D.C., fighting for sprouts. There is a major push to sterilize, process, homogenize, pasteurize, and—if it breathes—give it antibiotics proactively. This is contrary to what this book is about. This book is about eating fresh, natural, unprocessed food the way humans and other mammals have eaten since the beginning of time. The research around healthy gut flora and the microbiome is relatively new, and the positive impact of eating healthy foods on this biome is starting to be recognized. For fifteen years, I produced and provided raw and living food products to consumers. At Organic Avenue, we had to put a very scary warning on every cold-pressed juice sold, and every day, we made about fifty fresh, ripe, raw, untreated, unpasteurized products and sold millions of products over the years with an exceptional food safety and health track record.

I eat sprouts as often as possible and have no reservations about it. But of course the food you eat ultimately is your own decision. My recommendation is to be informed, follow the guidelines below, and go forth and sprout safely!

Cleanliness is key to sproutliness. When you are sprouting, you are dealing with nature and birthing of plants in the truest form. You are partnering with creation to activate dormant seeds into hyper-fast-growing plants. I like to compare seed sprouting to neonatal intensive care: the sprouts are fragile, with bacteria one of the biggest threats they face. For that reason, always wash your hands thoroughly or use food-safe gloves, and make sure everything your sprouts come into contact with, directly or indirectly, is perfectly clean. This means washing, rinsing, and either air-drying or towel-drying jars, trays, and other containers, countertops, utensils, and even the refrigerator and sink. I regularly spray my sink with a nontoxic, all-purpose disinfectant and cleaning agent. It's a good idea to sterilize your equipment periodically as well; use a similar practice to sterilizing baby bottles. Boiling or sterilizing agents such as hydrogen peroxide will do the job well. Place your sprouting equipment in a large pot, add enough water to cover all the equipment, and watch out for air bubbles. Bring the water to a boil and boil rapidly for five minutes. Turn off the heat and allow the water to cool down. Wash your hands again before handling the equipment.

Your number-one adversary to safe and scrumptious sprouts is mold. In most cases, when you think your seeds are sporting mold, you are actually seeing "root hairs," which look like fuzz around the seeds. This is normal, and the root hairs will disappear when you wash the seeds.

To prevent mold, first make sure you are using fresh seeds and that your sprouting equipment has been cleaned and sterilized. Always properly wash, drain, and rinse your seeds to keep them fresh and use room-temperature or slightly colder water, never hot water. Do not store the sprouting equipment in cabinets or under the sink; they need air.

In the event that your sprouts do have mold, that mold mostly likely will not be pathological but rather will be similar to the mold that grows on old bread—unsightly, perhaps, but when removed, the rest of the loaf or batch is not affected. Nonetheless, it's best to compost or trash that batch, sterilize the equipment, and start over.

Adding a sanitizing agent to your initial soaking water will help protect your seeds from mold and promote optimal unhindered growth. This is not a requirement, but it is an added measure to ensure the safety of your seeds, in particular if you're not using organic seeds or seeds not specifically designed for sprouting.

These are the sanitizing agents to choose from:

3.5 PERCENT FOOD-GRADE HYDROGEN PEROXIDE: Add five tablespoons per quart of water

PERACETIC ACID: Add four teaspoons per quart of water

CITROBIO: Add one-half teaspoon per quart of water

GRAPEFRUIT SEED EXTRACT: Add two drops per quart of water

Always dilute your agent, and be careful to avoid contact with skin and eyes. See Resources (pages 233–234) for where to find sanitizing agents.

Choose a Sprouting Method

Sprouting equipment has evolved considerably since I set out to sprout twenty-five years ago with a glass jar, cheesecloth, and a rubber band, but the fundamentals haven't changed. We're still attempting the same thing that humans have been doing since the beginning of time: to mimic Mother Nature and create an environment that will awaken the plant within. One of the amazing things about sprouting is that you can start with tools that you already have at home; it's an incredibly easy entry into DIY that anyone can accomplish. And if you're worried that it won't work for you, remember that it's not *about* you. The seed's destiny is to sprout, and without human intervention, the plant will replicate and multiply itself through its seeds.

The primary means to sprout today are jars, bags, tubes,

baskets/bowls, sprouting trays, and semiautomatic sprouters. I will cover them all here, along with setups for sprouting grasses and sunflower seeds in trays and special setups for gelatinous seeds like chia, arugula, and basil.

Most seeds will sprout with any method, whereas others are pickier. For example, lentils can be sprouted by any method, but tiny broccoli sprouts might get stuck in a hemp or muslin bag (but still will sprout with a little TLC) or fall through the large holes of a colander, and wheatgrass requires a porous tray. See the chart on pages 102–105 to pick the right method for your chosen seeds.

A BANG FOR YOUR BUCK AND YOUR BELLY

It's fascinating to picture how the seeds you plant will grow and take up so much more space relative to where they started as dormant seeds. For example, if you start with just one tablespoon of broccoli seeds, you will end up with about two cups of broccoli sprouts. Think about that exponential increase in volume and the room it will take up in your stomach. You wouldn't even notice eating one tablespoon of broccoli seeds, yet you will be fully satiated after snacking on a full two cups of sprouts in one sitting. For anyone who thinks they can't afford to eat organic, check out the math:

ORGANIC BROCCOLI SEEDS = $33 per pound of dry seeds, or about $2.10 per ounce
1 ounce (¼ cup) of dry seeds yields 8 cups broccoli sprouts
Bottom line: Broccoli sprouts cost about 30 cents per cup
ORGANIC MUNG BEANS = $7 per pound of dry beans, or about 45 cents per ounce
1 cup of dry mung beans = 3.75 ounces = $1.64

1 cup of dry mung beans yields 2 cups mung bean sprouts (the mature sprout with the long tail; immature mung bean sprouts will give a lesser yield)

Bottom line: Mung bean sprouts cost about 41 cents per cup

SHOPPING FOR SPROUTS IN THE STORE

For my first organic business, Organic Avenue, we made fifty or so fresh plant-based dishes every day across our ten retail stores in New York City. We used to have a sprout guy. He'd drive down from upstate New York in a truck to deliver sprouts to our loft. Until the sprout guy becomes as commonplace as the milkman of yore, the best place to shop for sprouts is the farmers' market. If that's not an option, go for a trusted natural food store or supermarket, and always abide by the sell-by or use-by dates. I wouldn't purchase a package of sprouts that has less than three or four days of shelf life left on it. While some smaller shops and co-ops may have a direct grower-to-market relationship, many times sprouts go through a bit of a journey—from the grower to a distributor, then to the market's warehouse, to the back room of the market—before making their way to the produce aisle. It could take days from the time they are harvested and packed until they end up on the shelf.

Look for bright, clean, crisp-looking sprouts with a sturdy structure. They should be the color of the seed or bean plus a white shoot. If they look mealy, show signs of browning or yellowing, or are stuck together, do not buy them. It goes without saying, but I'll say it anyway: Never buy sprouts with mold on them! See pages 249–250 for more on food safety concerns.

Sprouting in Glass Jars

Once I started sprouting, I would collect and save every glass jar that passed through my kitchen. I don't buy a lot of packaged food, but the things that I do buy, like coconut yogurt and sauerkraut, generally come in glass jars. A simple glass mason jar is a great option to get started, and it's space-effective, as soaking and sprouting both happen in the same jar. The only real requirement for a glass jar is that it has a wide mouth for maximum air circulation and easy access to the sprouts inside. Jars are perfect for most seeds, except when you want to grow a shoot or microgreen, such as with sunflower or wheatgrass, or gelatinous seeds such as arugula, flax, or chia.

> **TIP:** Mason jars can be found at hardware stores for a very small investment, or search them out at yard sales for a song. Vintage glassware will make your sprout setup Insta-worthy (show me yours @dougevans). Replace the tops of anything previously used, run the jars through the dishwasher, and they will be good as new.

I love looking at the seeds soaking in the water, and I typically have at least a dozen glass jars dominating my countertop at any given time. You might want to start your sprouting venture with a single glass jar, but don't be surprised to suddenly find your kitchen transformed into a mini sprout farm. Thoroughly wash your jars after you've grown and eaten your sprouts.

WHAT YOU NEED TO SPROUT IN A GLASS JAR:

Seeds

Measuring cup and spoons

Glass jar (a two-quart jar will give you ample room to grow a wide range of treasures)

Sanitizing agent (optional)

Screen (a dedicated plastic or stainless steel lid fitted with a screen [see below], cheesecloth, muslin, or an organic cotton sheet)

1. Inspect your bounty of seeds, and remove any broken, discolored, or damaged seeds.

2. Measure the amount of seeds required for your jar (see the chart on pages 102–105), and put them in the jar.

3. Wash the seeds very thoroughly.

4. Add water to cover (include a sanitizing agent in your soaking water as an extra precaution, if you like; see page 124), and let soak for two to three minutes.

5. Put on a lid fitted with a screen (see sidebar) or other cover and drain.

6. Rinse, cover with fresh water (without the sanitizing agent), and let soak for another two to three minutes, then drain again. Take this as an opportunity to be fully present and engaged in this life-affirming process.

7. Top your seeds off with water. A ratio of 3:1 water to seeds is a good standard rule. For example, if you are

using ¼ cup of seeds, add ¾ cup of water. Gently agitate the jar, and push down any floaters with a spoon.

8. Soak the seeds for five to eight hours depending on the seeds (see pages 102–105) at room temperature. Drain.

9. Store the jar in a cool, dark place at a 70-degree angle to ensure that residual water drains out (make sure there's a vessel underneath to catch that water). How to find a 70-degree angle? Start with upside down, which is 90 degrees, then point the mouth of the jar in the direction of six o'clock, but stop a little before so it lands at five o'clock (so it's almost upside down but at a slight angle). To achieve that angle, you could set your jar into a dedicated sprouting jar stand (see Resources, pages 233–234), a bowl, or the groove of a wooden carving board. Anything that will elevate your jar to 70 degrees will work—get creative!

10. Rinse and strain the seeds two or three times a day. Be gentle, and use this as a sacred time. You are basically the midwife to these seeds. Remember that your seeds are alive and fragile. Coddle them. If you shake, squeeze, scrape, or otherwise dis your budding sprouts, you could crush them or break the sprouts off the seeds prematurely and spoil the bunch.

11. When the tails get about one inch long (it will vary on a seed-by-seed basis—chickpea sprouts may be shorter than broccoli sprouts, for example) and you start to see leaves forming and splitting, your sprouts are ready to be harvested. Place the jar in a bright part

of the room with natural light for a few hours, but not in direct sunlight (direct sunlight will wilt if not kill your sprouts), for your sprouts to develop their vibrant green color.

12. After harvesting your sprouts, you can place them in a large bowl and cover them with water to separate the sprouts from stray seeds and shells. The sprouts should stay at the bottom, and the strays and shells will float to the top and can easily be strained away. Dry them in a salad spinner to remove excess water. This step is optional; I personally like to eat the stray seeds.

13. Store your sprouts directly in the jar with a standard airtight lid, or transfer them to another container or a zip-top bag and refrigerate them for up to one week. Rinse them once every two or three days and then strain very well to keep them fresh. (If you're storing the sprouts in a bag, dump them in a colander every two or three days, wet them down, drain them thoroughly, rinse the bag, and then return them to the bag.)

A FORK IN THE ROAD

When leafy salad sprouts have reached their full height, you have hit a fork in the road. You can eat your sprouts now, store them in the refrigerator, or expose them to a little sunlight and watch how their yellow leaves magically go through photosynthesis and form healthy green leaves. The chlorophyll that's produced at this step is the icing on the cake that gives your sprouts their beautiful green color.

CHOOSING THE RIGHT COVER FOR YOUR JAR

If you are sprouting in mason jars, you can purchase dedicated plastic or stainless steel screen lids to cover them with. These allow you to easily strain the water after soaking (see Resources, pages 233–234). Note that most screens only work with widemouthed mason jars.

Make sure to choose a strainer that has a smaller screen than the seed itself. I can say that with confidence, because I have underestimated many times. I used to love straining in one particular colander, but the first time I set out to sprout tiny celery seeds, about 50 percent went right through the colander and down the drain. At least those seeds were not lost in vain, as the water from my faucet directly waters a lovely creosote about ten feet from my house. Screens typically come in fine (for tiny sprouts like broccoli), medium (for lentil-size sprouts), and coarse (for large legumes like peas and chickpeas). Look for sets of the three. As your sprouts grow, you may switch up to a screen with a larger opening to maximize air circulation.

An alternative to the dedicated screen is a piece of

unbleached cheesecloth, muslin, a new undyed organic cotton pillowcase cut to size, or even pantyhose or an unused organic sock; hold it in place with the jar's ring if you have one or a rubber band. If you want to sprout on a large scale like I do, try using a five-gallon pail and secure the top with a pillowcase. You could feed your whole block!

Special Setups for Chia and Other Gelatinous Seeds

Gelatinous or mucilaginous seeds include chia, flax, arugula, basil, onion, and watercress. They are substantially different from other seeds in that as soon as they are immersed in water, they start to form a gel. This is great for chia pudding, but for sprouting, you don't want to get them too wet. Your sprouting platform for gelatinous seeds includes a hemp sprouting bag (you sprout *outside* the bag), a sprouting medium, an unbleached paper towel, or a terra-cotta clay sprouter (see Resources, pages 233–234). Distribute seeds evenly so that they touch but don't overlap across the surface. Keep at room temperature away from direct sunlight. Spray the entire surface with water from a spray bottle, making sure all the seeds are wet. Spray again after one hour, and continue to spray them multiple times a day for the first two to three days. If you are in a dry environment, loosely cover them with a clear plastic container upside down without a lid or plastic bag to create a greenhouse effect for the first two to three days to retain moisture. Continue to spray them at least two times a day. It will be exciting to watch them grow! Harvest them when they are between a half inch and two inches, in seven to fourteen days. They will keep in a covered jar in the refrigerator for up to one week.

Of course, you could sprout chia (and actually *any* gelatinous seeds) using a good old Chia Pet, and you get to have fun sprouting hair out of a host of adorable animals or even the head of a U.S. president. Unlike the methods described above, Chia Pets actually call for making a gel out of the seeds and spreading it over the figure.

Sprouting in Bags

If you are serious about air circulating around your little friends, you will love the sprouting bag method. The sprouting bag is a universal sprouting tool. It's very effective for several reasons, predominantly because of the air circulation it affords and the closer simulation to the environment in which a seed would naturally germinate in nature. A sprouting bag is more forgiving than a jar because it allows the sprouts to breathe and drain on all sides. If you are agile and crafty, you could sprout just about anything in or on a sprout bag. You can even grow gelatinous seeds, such as arugula, chia, and flax, using the bag method—they actually grow on the *outside* of the bag (see pages 132–133).

Sprouting bags, typically made from hemp or muslin, or nut milk bags that serve double duty for your sprouts, cost between five and fifteen dollars. Or you can make your own out of an undyed organic cotton pillowcase or cheesecloth. Just be forewarned that your kitchen may start looking like an organic co-op with bags hanging all over the place and pots or bowls underneath to catch the water! I love the look, but if that's not your thing, the jar method or a mix of the two is the way to go. Some people sprout everything in bags, while other people will just use them for legumes and grains. Rinse your bag in water with a sanitizing agent (page 124) mixed into it before sprouting in it. Rinse it in hot water in between uses and hang it up to dry—set it out in the sun to speed up the process.

WHAT YOU NEED TO SPROUT IN A BAG:

Seeds

Measuring cup and spoons

Glass jar or bowl (for soaking your seeds)

Sanitizing agent (optional)

Screen *(see pages 131–132) or fine-mesh strainer*

Hemp or muslin sprouting bag *(a cloth nut milk bag also will work)*

1. Inspect your bounty of seeds, and remove any broken, discolored, or damaged seeds.
2. Measure the amount of seeds required for your jar (see the chart on pages 102–105).
3. Wash the seeds very thoroughly.
4. Add water to cover (include a sanitizing agent in your soaking water as an extra precaution, if you like; see page 124) and let soak for two to three minutes.

5. Put on a lid fitted with a screen and drain, or strain through a fine-mesh strainer.

6. Rinse, cover with fresh water (without the sanitizing agent), and let soak for another two to three minutes, then drain again. Take this as an opportunity to be fully present and engaged in this life-affirming process.

7. Top your seeds off with water. A ratio of 3:1 water to seeds is a good standard rule. For example, if you are using ¼ cup of seeds, add ¾ cup of water. Gently agitate the jar, and push down any floaters with a spoon.

8. Soak the seeds for five to eight hours depending on the seeds (see pages 102–105) at room temperature. Drain.

9. Transfer the seeds into your sprouting bag, and either submerge the sealed bag underwater in a bowl or pot or place it under your water source for one to two minutes, until the seeds and bag are fully wet.

10. Pull the drawstring closed. Do not put the sprouting bag on a flat surface as you would a glass jar. Instead, hang the bag over the sink or a bowl to catch the water that drips out. A bamboo or steel banana holder will handily hold two or three bags; you also could set up an A-frame countertop clothes dryer on your counter or run a clothesline across your kitchen to hang multiple bags from.

11. Rinse, lightly massage (to keep the sprouts from attaching to the bag and each other), and drain the

seeds two or three times a day. Be gentle, and use this as a sacred time. You are basically the midwife to these seeds. Remember that your seeds are alive and fragile. Coddle them. If you shake, squeeze, scrape, or otherwise dis your budding sprouts, you could crush them or break the sprouts off the seeds prematurely and spoil the bunch. Don't wring the sprout bag like you would wring out a shirt!

12. When the tails grow to about a half inch, it's time to open the bag. Fold the bag down like you would cuff your jeans, and invite your sprouts to take their first glimpse of daylight. You will no longer be hanging the bag; instead, form the bag into a bowl shape and sit the bag directly on a plate. Instead of rinsing your sprouts, simply hydrate them two or three times a day using a spray bottle or the sprayer from your sink to simulate a rain shower.

13. When you start to see leaves forming and splitting, your sprouts are ready to be harvested. Place the bag in a bright part of the room with natural light for a few hours, but not in direct sunlight (direct sunlight will wilt if not kill your sprouts) for your sprouts to develop their vibrant green color.

14. After harvesting your sprouts, you can place them in a large bowl and cover them with water to separate the sprouts from stray seeds and shells. The sprouts should stay at the bottom, and the strays and shells will float to the top and can easily be strained away. Dry them

in a salad spinner to remove excess water. This step is optional; I personally like to eat the strays.

15. Store your sprouts directly in the bag or transfer them to another container or a zip-top bag and refrigerate them for up to one week. Rinse them once every two or three days, and strain very well to keep them fresh. (If you're storing the sprouts in a zip-top bag, dump them in a colander every two or three days, wet them down, drain them thoroughly, rinse the bag, and then return them to the bag.)

SPROUTING SMALLER SEEDS IN BAGS

Although sprouting bags traditionally are used for legumes and grains, they can be used for smaller sprouts such as broccoli as well. For best results, after a day or two of sprouting, place the bag on a plate and form the bag into a cylinder shape with a flat bottom. Roll the bag down so light can get in there and the sprouts can grow up. At this point, you are treating the bag like a bowl or a tray and using the trusty old spray bottle to hydrate them.

Junkyard Dog

If you think about the amount of random stuff on the planet or in your kitchen, it can be overwhelming. Why not take your personal overabundance as an opportunity to create your own customized sprouter! Virtually every container that has food shipped in it has to be approved food-safe. Non-BPA plastic containers, lids, and food-grade packaging can go into your sprouting toolshed to become platforms for sprouting. Make sure you wash them well and recycle them if they get damaged.

Sprouting tubes are like jars but with the bonus of airflow from both ends. To make a sprouting tube, get a piece of clear, food-grade plastic three or four inches in diameter and wash it well. Place a piece of cheesecloth, muslin, pantyhose, or unbleached organic cotton cloth on either end and fasten with a rubber band or kitchen string. Follow the instructions for sprouting in jars (see pages 127–130).

Sprouting baskets were very popular in the hippie generation of the '60s and '70s, when you'd find untreated bamboo or natural fiber baskets hanging everywhere. Nowadays, it's hard to find a basket that's woven tightly enough so the seeds initially won't fall through, so you can employ a hybrid method: Line a basket with a piece of fabric or a sprouting bag. The basket will keep the shape of the sprouts and is porous so the water will drain and the sprouts can grow up vertically. Most baskets today are more decorative than functional, so if you can't confirm that your basket has not been treated with chemicals, do not use this method.

Colanders are easy and handy, as most households have one for straining pasta or rice or rinsing beans or vegetables. Their design enables water to flow so the seeds don't sit in water as they sprout. Make sure the holes are small enough to prevent the seeds from falling through.

Plastic bottles and jugs can be cut to your desired length and shape. Punch or cut holes in them to create drainage. These come in handy when you're experimenting with new seeds or you want to initiate a second or third batch of the same seed and your primary containers are full. They also make the kitchen look very interesting!

Plastic clamshells that have been used to sell berries, greens, or sprouts can be repurposed. Line the side that has holes with an unbleached paper towel, add seeds that have been soaked and drained, and spray them with water two or three times a day.

Semiautomatic Sprouters

We are living in the most exciting times when it comes to technology. We can turn on light switches with our iPhones and flip a switch in our garage to put our sprinklers on autopilot and take care of the lawn for a whole season. Automation has come to the sprout world as well. There are a lot of commercially available sprouting machines on the market today. Conceptually, they are very good ideas, but in practical terms, they still require some work. There are two fundamental types as of this writing, both with water sprayed over the sprouts on a programmed schedule.

One is a round basket that sits over a reservoir; it has a center sprinkler like a fountain that spins around and sprays the water on top of the seeds as they sprout. It's fascinating to watch the hard little seeds seemingly magically grow into mature sprouts. My fundamental concern with these is that they collect the water after it has been sprayed and then respray it, in effect reusing the water. The instructions are to clean the automatic sprouter after each harvest, but I believe that the sprouts like fresh water best and that the water should be changed as much as once or twice a day. If you're with me on that, then you are better off using one of the low-tech sprouting methods. Many people swear by automatic sprouters, though, and if it makes it a little easier and you are satisfied with the results, go for it.

There's another type of automatic sprouter that has both a water source and a drain. This is very cool and addresses my concerns with the ones that recirculate water. If you are new to sprouting and are up for investing $50–$250, this could be a good way to get started. I got very excited the first time I used one of these because it did what it said it was going to do. But be aware that there is some cleaning involved after each cycle, and for those of us obsessed with food safety (we all should be!), it is a process.

Sprouting in Trays

This is what the professionals do (aside from the massive bath-tubs filled with mung bean sprouts that you will find in New York's Chinatown), and you can too. Every type of seed can be sprouted and grown effectively in a tray. You can purchase a dedicated sprouting tray, or if you have a spare cafeteria-type tray, you can drill some holes in the bottom and use it as your DIY sprout tray. All you need is a flat surface with holes and a border to contain the sprouts and something as simple as an unbleached paper towel, coconut coir, or hemp or burlap fabric as the growing medium. At a restaurant supply store, I recently saw beautiful stainless steel trays with the perfect-size holes that fit right into a stainless steel baker's rack. I am putting that on my wish list for sure. You can also make inexpensive multitier sprouting trays with holes in the bottom for drainage for stackable sprouting (see Resources, pages 233–234).

WHAT YOU NEED TO SPROUT IN A TRAY:
Seeds
Measuring cups and spoons
Glass bowl or jar (for soaking your seeds)
Sanitizing agent (optional)
Sprouting tray (see Resources, pages 233–234)
Unbleached paper towels
Spray bottle

1. Inspect your bounty of seeds, and remove any broken, discolored, or damaged seeds.
2. Measure the amount of seeds required for your tray (see the chart on pages 102–105).
3. Wash the seeds very thoroughly.
4. Add water to cover (include a sanitizing agent in your

soaking water as an extra precaution, if you like; see page 124) and let soak for two to three minutes.

5. Put on a lid fitted with a screen and drain, or strain through a fine-mesh strainer.

6. Rinse, cover with fresh water (without the sanitizing agent), and let soak for another two to three minutes, then drain again. Take this as an opportunity to be fully present and engaged in this life-affirming process.

7. Top your seeds off with water. A ratio of 3:1 water to seeds is a good standard rule. For example, if you are using ¼ cup of seeds, add ¾ cup of water. Push down any floaters.

8. Soak the seeds for five to eight hours depending on the seeds (see pages 102–105) at room temperature. Drain.

9. Wash your sprouting tray (to sanitize it, spray it with a sanitizing agent or dip it in boiling hot water). You want it nice and clean, as befits a proper host for your seeds in their early intensive-care stage.

10. Line your sprouting tray with a double layer of unbleached paper towel.

11. Pour the drained seeds onto the paper towel, and spread them out in a very tight single layer. Did you ever see the video from the rush hour trains in Japan with people in the station whose sole responsibility is getting as many people onto the train as possible without piling them on top of each other? You want those seeds tight, but you also want them in a single layer.

12. Using a spray bottle or the sprayer from your sink (if your water is filtered), mist the tray in a methodical

pattern to ensure that 100 percent of the seeds get watered. Cover with an opaque lid; this can be a section of a black garbage bag, a dishwasher tray, or even a light plastic lunch plate. Your germinating seeds prefer darkness to simulate what it's like to be in the earth or the intestinal tract of an animal.

13. Spray two or three times a day. The seeds are counting on you to keep them hydrated!

14. When tails start to grow, cover the tray with a clear tray or clear heavy-duty plastic liner (typically used for recycling). At this stage, the seeds like natural daylight but do not dig direct sunlight.

15. Continue to water two to three times a day. When the seeds grow shoots and leaves, depending on the seeds (three to ten inches), you can now begin to harvest by cutting them as close to the root level as possible. Every seed is different, and some sprouts will continue to grow. The seed fundamentally contains enough nutrition to get you to this stage. If you don't harvest at this point, you will need to fertilize them with a fertilizer such as liquid kelp (see Resources, pages 233–234).

16. To store your sprouts, transfer them to a container and cover, or place them in a zip-top bag and refrigerate them for up to one week. Rinse them once every two or three days, and strain very well to keep them fresh. (If you're storing the sprouts in a bag, dump them in a colander every two or three days, wet them down, drain them thoroughly, rinse the bag, and then return them to the bag.)

Sprouting Grasses in Trays

Though wheatgrass has become the most well-known and available of the cereal grasses, most grasses, from barley grass, oat grass, spelt grass, to rye grass, are similar and can be sprouted, grown, and used interchangeably. For the purpose of this section, I will reference wheatgrass, but you can use your preferred grass. Most wheat seeds found in health food stores are intended for bread baking rather than sprouting. For best results, purchase directly from a source that sells dedicated sprouting seeds (see Resources, pages 233–234). See page 95 to learn about the uses and benefits of wheatgrass and other grasses.

WHAT TO DO WITH GRASSES

Cows have four stomachs and can chew on grass all day. Since we have only one stomach, the preferred method of extracting the nutrition from grasses is juicing. You can purchase a dedicated manual wheatgrass juicer for under $100, and that will do just fine. Alternatively, if you are feeling feral, you could chew and chew and chew and then spit out the indigestible cellulose. I like to take a handful of wheatgrass blades with me to chew on a hike. It does wonders for my teeth, gums, breath, and digestion. The hardest part is remembering that I have only one stomach and not to swallow the fiber!

WHAT YOU NEED TO SPROUT GRASSES IN TRAYS:

1½ to 2 cups dry wheatgrass, barley grass, oat grass, spelt grass, or rye grass seeds (this will make enough for three or four two-ounce shots of grass to drink)

Measuring cups and spoons

Glass bowl or jar (for soaking your seeds)

Sanitizing agent (optional)

13 × 19-inch sprouting tray (see Resources, pages 233–234)

Unbleached paper towels or organic soil (see sidebar, pages 146–147)

Spray bottle

To soak the seeds:

1. Inspect your bounty of seeds, and remove any broken, discolored, or damaged seeds.

2. Measure the seeds and wash them very thoroughly.

3. Place the seeds in a jar, add water to cover (include a sanitizing agent in your soaking water as an extra precaution, if you like; see page 124), and let soak for two to three minutes.

4. Put on a lid fitted with a screen and drain, or strain through a fine-mesh strainer.

5. Rinse, cover with fresh water (without the sanitizing agent), and let soak for another two to three minutes, then drain again. Take this as an opportunity to be fully present and engaged in this life-affirming process.

6. Top your seeds off with water. A ratio of 3:1 water to seeds is a good standard rule. For example, if you are using ¼ cup of seeds, add ¾ cup of water. Push down any floaters.

7. Soak the seeds for five to eight hours depending on the seeds (see pages 102–105) at room temperature. Drain.

8. Wash and sanitize your sprouting tray. You want it nice and clean, as befits a proper host for your seeds in their early intensive-care stage.

> **TIP:** *Use the spray bottle that you'll use to water your "lawn," a.k.a. the wheatgrass blades (or any soaking seeds, for that matter), to saturate floaters that don't want to stay submerged. Saturating your seeds primes them for optimal sprouting success.*

SOIL AND SOIL ALTERNATIVES

I recommend a "loose and light" nutrient-dense organic soil in a 1:1 ratio of peat moss to topsoil. *Loose and light* means the soil has large particles and is loose and easy to work with. You can find this type of soil at most garden supply stores. Soil gardening requires more attention than other avenues of sprouting, as the soil can play host to mold more easily than soil-free gardening.

If you opt to go soil-free, you have several options to consider:

Unbleached paper towel: This is the most economical option and does a very acceptable job, and the whole thing goes right into the compost after harvesting.

Burlap: This is an affordable option that you can buy new or maybe even get for free from your local coffee roaster. Grasses do really well on burlap.

Coco coir: Composed of 100 percent coco fiber from coconut husk, it does a great job of staying moist. Coco coir gets great results, especially over burlap and unbleached paper towels.

Hemp mats: Hemp is a very versatile crop and performs well in many situations. The hemp acts like a mulch and retains water well.

TO GROW THE SEEDS:

To grow the seeds in soil:

Fill your sprouting tray with ⅟₁₆ inch of soil and disperse the seeds evenly across the tray so they touch snuggly. To simulate growing outside, place a paper towel over the seeds and spray it until it's wet, or top with a dusting of soil. It's important to distribute the seeds evenly, snug but not stacked on top of one another. If seeds were strangers on the subway in New York City, they would be packed uncomfortably close!

To grow the seeds without soil:

Cover your sprouting tray with a double layer of moistened, unbleached paper towel. Paper towels provide a soft bed for the seeds to hang out on and make cleanup a jiffy. (And they are a favorite for the worms in the compost!) Cover the paper towels with your seeds, taking care to distribute the seeds evenly. The seeds should be close, kissing each other.

DAYS 1 TO 3

These three days are of utmost importance. It is vital to remain vigilant over your sprouts, as the degree to which you dedicate yourself will determine sprouting success. As the seed matures, it will be more tolerant, but in the first few days, it absolutely needs water twice a day. Fill up your spray bottle with fresh water each day, and spray the seeds with water twice daily for about thirty seconds. Cover with an opaque lid; this can be a section of a black garbage bag, a dishwasher tray, or even light plastic lunch plates. You are looking to create a dark and damp environment to nurture your sleeping seedlings until they begin to shoot out and sprout. When the grass is growing evenly on Day 3 (if it isn't, wait another day or two), remove the opaque cover and replace it with a clear plastic bag, another seed tray, or a light, clear dedicated cover that you can find in the store with the sprouting trays to form a little green-house, allowing natural light and air to reach the green shoots.

DAY 4

Green growth should be evident (if it's not, continue watering and rinsing), and it's time to closely examine your setup for mold. Do not be alarmed if mold is present, as it can easily be remedied. If you see signs of mold, rinse your sprouts and soak them for two to three minutes in water enriched with a sanitizing agent (see page 124), as this will further oxygenate the sprouts and prevent prevalence of mold.

DAY 5

Continue to mist the shoots twice daily and monitor for mold. If you see signs of mold, remove it as instructed for Day 4.

DAYS 6 TO 8

The apex of the journey is over. The rest of the ride is smooth sailing. The root systems will continue to develop, and the grass will be growing evenly. Once the grass reaches a height of one inch, remove the clear cover. This will allow air to circulate, oxygenating your sprouts and gearing them for a great harvest. At this stage, as with every stage prior, check for mold! Continue to spray with water twice daily to keep the seeds from drying and dying.

DAYS 10 TO 14

Happy harvesting! Once shoots of grass reach the sweet spot of six to twelve inches, it's game on and time to juice. If you let them get taller than twelve inches, it's gonna be out of control, like my hair. Harvest the shoots using a knife or scissors. Try harvesting some at six inches and some more the next day and ideally finish the tray by the time they reach twelve inches.

TIP: *I recently purchased a pair of ceramic scissors and thought, Where have you been my whole life?*

Cut the shoots just above the seed bed and compost the soil. If you plan on juicing, two ounces of wheatgrass blades yield a little over one ounce of juice. Store trimmed grass refrigerated in green plastic produce bags (available in most health food stores, or see Resources, pages 233–234), where they will keep for ten to twenty days. I like to get my first juice in on the day that I harvest.

Begin a batch every three to four days, as this will keep rotation moving and provide a robust harvest!

Growing Microgreens

Microgreens are the tiny edible form of nutrient-dense green leafy vegetables, herbs, or other plants that are in between sprouts and their mature vegetable counterparts. They range in size from one to two inches tall, including the stem and leaves. The flavors are full and more advanced than sprouts but not as intense as the fully mature plant. There is really nothing new about microgreens other than the label they acquired in the mid-1990s. Plants always go through the microgreen stage en route to becoming a full-grown plant; they just stop early. This is a really good thing to do, because not only are microgreens palate pleasers, the research has found that they actually contain more vitamins, antioxidants, and minerals than the full-size plant (as they grow, they take up essential elements and nutrients from the soil, but they are also increasing the fiber, thereby diluting the nutrient-to-mass ratio). Growing microgreens is just as easy as growing sprouts, but they take a little more time and a slightly different set of tools. In the Sprout

Primer, I call out basil and celery to be grown specifically as microgreens, as they are difficult to sprout, but just about any vegetable seed that can sprout can continue to grow into a microgreen (or fully grown plant).

WHAT YOU NEED TO GROW MICROGREENS:
Seeds
Measuring cups and spoons
Glass jar or bowl (for soaking your seeds)
Sanitizing agent (optional; see page 124)
Sprouting tray (see Resources, pages 233–234)
Organic soil (see sidebar, pages 146–147) or unbleached paper towels
Spray bottle

1. Inspect your bounty of seeds, and remove any broken, discolored, or damaged seeds.
2. Measure your seeds and wash them very thoroughly.
3. Place the seeds in a jar, add water to cover (include a sanitizing agent in your soaking water as an extra precaution, if you like; see page 124), and let soak for two to three minutes.
4. Put on a lid fitted with a screen and drain, or strain through a fine-mesh strainer.
5. Rinse, cover with fresh water (without the sanitizing agent), and let soak for another two to three minutes,

then drain again. Take this as an opportunity to be fully present and engaged in this life-affirming process.

6. Top your seeds off with water. A ratio of 3:1 water to seeds is a good standard rule. For example, if you are using ¼ cup of seeds, add ¾ cup of water. Push down any floaters with a spoon.

7. Soak the seeds for five to eight hours depending on the seeds (see pages 102–105) at room temperature. Drain.

8. Wash and sanitize your sprouting tray (see page 142). You want it nice and clean, as befits a proper host for your seeds in their early intensive-care stage.

9. Fill your sprouting tray with one to two inches of soil, or line it with a double layer of moistened, unbleached paper towel or a coconut or hemp sprouting medium. Paper towels provide a soft bed for the seeds to hang out on and make cleanup a jiffy. Disperse the seeds evenly across the tray.

10. Cover with a damp cotton cloth or paper towel. This will keep the seeds moist, as they grow best in a dark and damp environment.

11. Over the next twenty-four to forty-eight hours, spray the seeds twice a day.

12. After twenty-four to forty-eight hours, the seeds will sprout tails. At this point, if you are sprouting in soil, sprinkle the seeds with soil and continue to spray twice a day, allowing the seeds to receive indirect light and plenty of air circulation.

13. Monitor the microgreens until they measure two to four inches in height. This will take anywhere from one to two weeks. Once they reach this optimal height, they are ready for harvest! If you are not ready to consume the microgreens, fear not; simply place the microgreens in the refrigerator to suspend their growth. I have not found a material difference in the height of microgreens grown in soil versus on paper towels. Every time you bring seeds to life, you're partnering with nature, and there will always be different variables, including weather, temperature, light, or batch of seeds.

Growing Sunflower Shoots and Pea Shoots

Driving down a country road, a field of sunflowers stand, their faces stretching tall toward the sun. The sunflower, *Helianthus,* a genus native to North America containing around seventy different species, possesses not only aesthetic beauty but outstanding health benefits as well. Harvesting sunflower seeds in a field may not be quite feasible, so I suggest sprouting seeds in your kitchen following this simple and straightforward method of harvesting health right in your own home. Sprouting sunflower seeds was a huge revelation to me, and sunflower sprouts have become my all-time favorite sprout for their superior flavor, texture, and chewiness.

Although it's the same seed, there is a distinct difference between hulled and unhulled seeds. For sprouting, I am referencing the seed with the black shell that may have a white line on it and that looks like birdseed, not the light gray seeds that are edible right out of the bag or can be soaked or sprouted and eaten like any other nut or seed. Sunflower seed shells must be washed meticulously.

Pea shoots are tender and delightful greens that are sweet and easy to chew. I have yet to meet anyone who didn't love them. (Pea sprouts, on the other hand, look like normal garden peas with a little tail and are packed with protein. They fall into the legume category like chickpeas and lentils and are sprouted as such.)

Sunflower shoots and pea shoots can be grown on paper towels (and if you're using paper towels, you don't even need a sprouting tray—you could use a baking sheet). If you have the time and space, soil provides comfort for the seeds to grow roots and shoots while providing additional minerals that will affect their flavor and nutrition.

WHAT YOU NEED TO GROW SHOOTS:

Seeds

Measuring cups and spoons

Glass jar or bowl (for soaking your seeds)

Sanitizing agent (optional; see page 124)

Sprouting tray (see Resources, pages 233–234)

Organic soil (see sidebar, page 146) **or unbleached paper towels**

Spray bottle

1. Inspect your bounty of seeds, and remove any broken, discolored, or damaged seeds.

2. Measure your seeds and wash them very thoroughly.

3. Place the seeds in a jar, add water to cover (include a sanitizing agent in your soaking water as an extra precaution, if you like; see page 124), and let soak for two to three minutes.

4. Put on a lid fitted with a screen and drain, or strain through a fine-mesh strainer.

5. Rinse, cover with fresh water (without the sanitizing agent), and let soak for another two to three minutes, then drain again. Take this as an opportunity to be fully present and engaged in this life-affirming process.

6. Top your seeds off with water. A ratio of 3:1 water to seeds is a good standard rule. For example, if you are using ¼ cup of seeds, add ¾ cup of water. Push down any floaters.

7. Soak the seeds for five to eight hours depending on the seeds (see pages 102–105) at room temperature. Drain.

8. Wash and sanitize your sprouting tray. You want it nice and clean, as befits a proper host for your seeds in their early intensive-care stage.

9. Fill your sprouting tray with one to two inches of soil, or line it with a double layer of moistened, unbleached paper towel or a coconut or hemp sprouting medium. Paper towels provide a soft bed for the seeds to hang

out on and make cleanup a jiffy. Disperse the seeds
evenly across the tray.

10. Cover with a damp cotton cloth or paper towel. This
will keep the seeds moist, as they grow best in a dark
and damp environment.

11. Over the next twenty-four to forty-eight hours, spray
the seeds twice a day.

12. After twenty-four to forty-eight hours, the sunflower
seeds will sprout tails. At this point, if you are
sprouting in soil, sprinkle the sprouts with soil and
continue to spray twice a day, allowing the seeds to
receive indirect light and plenty of air circulation.

13. Monitor the shoots until they measure two to four
inches in height. This will take anywhere from one to
two weeks. Once they reach this optimal height, they
are ready for harvest! If you are not ready to consume
the sprouts, fear not; simply place the shoots in the
refrigerator to suspend their growth. I have not found
a material difference in the height shoots grow in soil
versus on paper towels. Every time you sprout, you're
partnering with nature, and there are always different
variables, including weather, temperature, light, or
batch of seeds.

Set Out with a Plan

A failure to plan is a plan to fail. This is a common mantra I lived by both in the military and in my business career. Take a moment to develop a sprouting plan by writing down or imagining what your goals are; for example, to always have a garnish or salad topper at the ready for targeted nutrition or to make the recipes on pages 169–229. What's motivating you, and what kind of harvest and bounty would you like to receive? This will help you decide what equipment and seeds to buy, and when everything comes in, you are ready to rock and sprout. There are as many different sprouters as there are sprouts. Let's meet a one.

Jane the Junior Partner: "Her Doctor Planted Some Seeds"

Jane Wilson is a twenty-eight-year-old junior partner lawyer who works in a medium-size firm near Wall Street. Jane is a litigator and works many hours in and out of the office. She manages to run anywhere from two to four miles five to six days a week. She likes to take her weekends off, unless she traveled during the week and then uses the weekends to make up for the lost runs. She's a vegan for ethical and environmental reasons, but she eats a lot of processed vegan food. This could include commercially manufactured veggie burgers, brown rice pasta, bottled sauces, bread (she loves bread), and energy bars. She looks at food as fuel but also will pretty much eat anything as long as it's vegan. Although Jane has a steady running routine, she's doesn't eat the healthiest foods on a consistent basis. She likes salads and greens, but she also likes bread, comfort foods, starches, desserts, and wine. At her last visit to the doctor, the doctor said that she was in good health but the aches and pains and tiredness were a concern. Her doctor is a longtime advocate of healthy food and sprouting and "planted some seeds" in Jane's brain.

Jane did some searches online and was astounded at the amount of published literature on the benefits of sprouting and decided to stick her toe in the water.

She got off to a good start. She bought a book on sprouting, a one-pound bag of organic broccoli seeds with a guaranteed 90+ percent germination rate, and decided to use one of the many mason jars that she had in her dusty kitchen cabinets. Jane read the basic instructions on the sprout bag that said, "Place two tablespoons of seeds with three times as much water as the seeds. Soak overnight, put a piece of cheesecloth or a fine strainer over the jar and pour out the excess water, fill up the jar with water again and rinse." Jane made a cockamamie setup of placing the strainer over a half-gallon pot and turning the jar upside down with a dish towel over it to keep it dark. About three days later, Jane remembered that she had broccoli seeds in a jar sprouting. *Uh-oh.* She was met with a moldy, coagulated, lightly stinky mess.

Jane reread the instructions and realized her fatal mistake—she had not rinsed the seeds two or three times a day. She was candidly discouraged and a bit angry at herself. Jane decided to head out to the health food store, bought a five-ounce package of broccoli sprouts, and inhaled them in about a minute. Even though she was unsuccessful in her first attempt to sprout on her own, she still was eating broccoli sprouts and following the doctor's orders. She continued on with her plans for the night but committed to trying again.

She got home that night relatively late, but definitely not too late to soak some seeds. With the discipline of a trial lawyer, she reread the instructions and took notes on a Post-it pad . . .

1. Two parts seeds, six parts water
2. Soak overnight
3. Rinse and strain the excess water
4. Store in dark place or cover with a cloth
5. Order screen lid online, but use strainer to start with
6. Set calendar alerts on iPhone for two times a day
7. Speak to the seeds and marvel at their growth
8. Keep a log

Jane carefully and meticulously followed her instructions for the two tablespoons of broccoli seeds that she wanted to sprout. She kept notes, set her timer, and to her great relief and surprise, the seeds were sprouting, the shoots and leaves were healthy, and Jane even was inspired to give them some sunlight to make the leaves green. Jane was over the moon with her first successful batch of broccoli sprouts.

Activate Your Midas Touch

Sprouting is as much of an art as it is a science. Although the process is very simple on paper, when the seed meets the water, the results sometimes can be unpredictable. Your seeds are about to go through a complete metamorphic transmutation from a hard, dry, dormant plant to a plant that is alive and filled with an enormous amount of life force. Nature has perfected this process from the beginning of time, and when we germinate at home, we are acting like nature and must do our best to create an environment that is suitable and supportive of the seed's journey into a sprout. That's a lot of responsibility, but it becomes very easy with practice. The good news is that those seeds are alive and are designed by nature to sprout. That makes you and the seed very aligned. The seed wants to sprout, and you want the seed to sprout! Developing a Midas touch with sprouting is easier than you may think; it just takes a little practice.

Factors that come into play when sprouting include indoor temperature, water temperature, water pH, water solids, chemicals or minerals in the water, type of lighting (natural versus electric), type of seeds, source of seeds, age of seeds, how the seeds were stored, type of sprouting vessel, method of sprouting, amount of seeds in the process, amount of time soaking, number of times rinsing, how clean your sprouting environment is, how clean your sprouting vessel is, how much water you added, how much soil you used, and the relative humidity of the environment. Those are just a few of the considerations and decisions that will ultimately affect your successful sprouting. We are indeed dancing with Mother Nature in a complex environment called earth where seemingly anything can happen. How exciting! Here are some ways to ensure smooth sailing:

1. **Buy seeds designed to sprout.** Seriously make the effort to buy seeds that are organic and that are designed for sprouting. These will have the highest germination rate and give you the highest yield and least frustration.

2. **Read the instructions carefully and follow them even more carefully.** You will get much better results if you follow the recommended sprouting protocol. Seeds can easily be killed by drowning or lack of water, or they can become moldy or mealy if not properly rinsed and kept in the right environment. Observe the soaking protocol on a seed-by-seed basis with the right amount of time for each specific seed. Think of the old adage "You never have enough time to do it right, but you always have time to do it again." I remember the first time I bought a dresser from IKEA. I was hot to trot and tore everything open and just started assembling, screwing, and attaching while glancing occasionally at the instructions. It was a disaster. It turns out there were lots of screws and pegs that looked the same but were slightly different sizes. So after taking the whole thing apart, laying it out exactly as the manual described, and matching every part to the designated code, I was able to assemble the darn thing in a little over an hour. Screwing it up the first time took more than three hours. I love reading manuals now, and your sprouts will love you for setting out with a plan.

3. **Choose the ideal sprouting location.** Since we are creating an earthy environment inside our homes, we need to find the ideal spot with the right temperature and light and make sure to rinse two or three times a day. Is it absolutely necessary that you do this 100 percent of the time? The answer is yes. Imagine a baby in neonatal intensive care. Your seeds are your babies, and they are in an incubator and need a lot of

love and attention to survive. They have no one else to call on! If you take good care of them, they will take great care of you.

4. **Use a timer.** A timer will ensure that you are soaking the right amount of time, enough but not too much. I use a combination of timers, an alarm clock, and a Google calendar with reminders. It's very easy to miss a soak, rinse, or harvest. Setting up reminders that will keep you connected to your sprouts will make you both very happy.

5. **Make sure the seeds don't drown.** The seeds need water, but only so much. If the instructions say to soak for four hours but you leave them overnight, the seeds can get waterlogged and might not receive enough oxygen to germinate.

6. **Use spring water, distilled water, or filtered water for soaking, rinsing, and growing your seeds.** Read about my journey off the water grid on pages 119–121.

7. **Keep your sprouting area clean.** It's very important to take tender loving care of not just your sprouts but their environment. Maintain a consistent protocol for keeping your sprouting area clean. This means washing down the kitchen countertops, sinks, refrigerator, and all equipment that comes in contact with the sprouts. And don't forget your hands. I wash my hands as carefully as a doctor going into surgery. Food safety is extra important when it comes to sprouts. Read more on the subject on pages 249–251.

8. **Be flexible.** Know that things change from seed to seed. A general rule of thumb is that smaller

seeds germinate faster than larger seeds. Ambient temperature also affects the germination process. Some of us still talk about the seasons, but most people use either heating or air-conditioning all the time to keep the temperature at a comfy 69 degrees. Although I personally like to stress my system by going out in the cold without a jacket, sprouts generally will germinate faster in warmer environments than colder climes.

9. **Create a Sprout Captain's Log.** This has been an extremely helpful practice for me. This is exactly what you might think it will be: a log that you write on every time you enter your sprouting den. As you get more experienced, you can start to abbreviate, but in the beginning, you want to be thorough and as detailed as possible. Here is a clip from my log:

Doug the Sprout Captain's Log

Sunday, 3/3/2019 6:45 a.m.

- Rinsed the 3-day-old mung bean sprouts in the 2-quart glass jar.
- Spray-watered the 2-day-old tray of wheatgrass.
- Dipped the broccoli sprouts in the hemp sprout bag in water and hung them back up.
- Started a new batch of broccoli sprouts in a glass jar. ¼ cup of seeds and ¾ cup of water. Pushed down all the floaters and set a timer for 8 hours.
- Removed the cover from 3-day-old sunflower seeds that were about 1 inch tall and sprouting and moved to a lighter area in the kitchen.

That might seem like a lot to write, but you will be so grateful you did when you look back and want to do a similar batch or, more important, if things don't go as planned.

10. **Remember that you cannot recover, but you can always redo.** We're all human and make mistakes from time to time. But when it comes to sprouting, you cannot revive or recover your mistakes. It's okay. Seeds are relatively inexpensive, and within every adversity, every failure, every misstep lies a lesson. Therefore, if you make a mistake, or you even suspect you made a mistake, abort, and toss your attempt into the compost. Wash the equipment thoroughly and properly and start again. It's like a baby learning to walk. It will take time and practice, and before you know it, the kid is grown up and out of the house. In the beginning, you may ask yourself, *Will this seed ever germinate?!* Some seeds that look very similar to one another will have totally different germination times. For example, broccoli seeds start to germinate in two to four days, but celery seeds can take up to eighteen days. That's not a typographical error! Eighteen days of soaking, rinsing, wetting, spraying, praying, and moving around the kitchen until they sprout a little tail!

Congratulations . . . you are an official sprout farmer! Now it's time to get into the kitchen and turn your harvest into incredibly tasty creations, from smoothies to salads, soups, street food, and even dessert!

THE RECIPES

Sprouts as a Side Dish, Meal,
and Supplement All in One
Neat Little Package

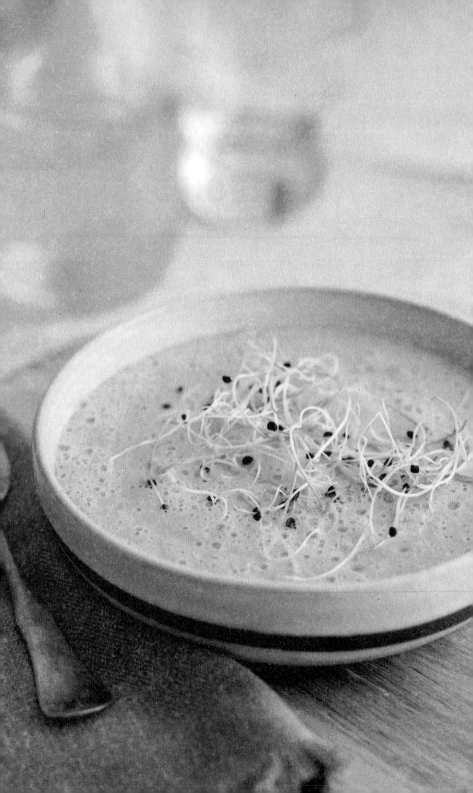

SPROUTS ARE THE pinnacle of plant-based cuisine. Add sprouts to your dishes and you radically raise the nutrition and flavor frequencies of your food. Go boldly by adding sprouts to salads and wraps or clandestinely by blending them into smoothies, pesto, salsa, and even dessert. With a slight shift in mind-set, your relationship with the food you eat will be transformed.

The flavors of sprouts are diverse, from mild alfalfa to bitter fenugreek, grassy garden pea, pungent onion, slightly sweet adzuki, and spicy radish. Mild mature mung bean sprouts have a high percentage of water, so they act as liquid nutrition in a number of the recipes, from smoothies to gazpacho. Consider the sprouts called for in each recipe as a jumping-off point, and take liberties to swap out what you have available; just generally stay within the same broad categories (e.g., swap clover for broccoli sprouts because they are both salad green sprouts, and swap chickpea for adzuki bean sprouts). Most of the recipes rely on the more common sprouts that can be found in grocery stores, such as mung bean, chickpea, lentil, broccoli, clover, and alfalfa, but feel free to swap or add in any DIY sprouts you might have going, from arugula to basil or watercress. Any recipe that calls for a blender will require a high-speed blender; sprouts are tough guys and need some extra muscle to break them down. A mini blender would come in handy for blending small amounts, such as for the Golden Tahini Dressing (page 216) or Green Pea Avocado Cream (page 217).

The recipes all fall into my preferred plant-based style: raw-food vegan. Sprouts really shine in their raw state (they tend to become a soggy, less nutritious mess when cooked), and that's how they are showcased here. Feel free to warm soups and cereals slightly, but just until warm to the touch so you retain their unprocessed and fresh flavor. If oil and salt are a concern to you, feel free to adjust the amounts or omit them. Note: The storage times for each dish assume freshly sprouted sprouts; if they have been around for any amount of time, subtract that amount from the total keeping time.

When in doubt, just add sprouts!

BEVERAGES AND BREAKFAST

SPROUTED ALMOND MILK

If you've made almond milk before, you probably soaked the almonds before blending them into milk. Sprouting after soaking takes your almond milk a step further by increasing enzyme activity and digestibility so you can get the most nutrition out of the nuts. It takes extra time, but very little extra effort, and you'll be hooked on the fresh, pure flavor DIY almond milk delivers! Note that almonds do not always grow a visible tail; don't fret, though, you've still unlocked their nutrition with the soak.

Makes 1 quart

1½ cups sprouted almonds
4 cups water

Combine the sprouted almonds and water in a blender and blend, starting on low speed and working your way up to high, until smooth, about 2 minutes. Strain through a nut milk bag or strainer lined with cheesecloth into a bowl. Squeeze on the pulp to extract all the liquid. Pour into a jar and refrigerate until ready to use. It will keep refrigerated for up to 4 days.

SUPER GREEN SPROUT SMOOTHIE

This smoothie is a deliciously drinkable source of protein, boasting more than 20 grams of protein plus bonus vitamins, minerals, phytochemicals, and lots of fiber. Sip this for breakfast and any day will be the best day ever!

Serves 1

½ cup unsweetened almond milk, preferably Sprouted
   Almond Milk (page 169)
3 tablespoons fresh lemon juice
2 cups (about 4 ounces) mature mung bean sprouts
4 ounces romaine lettuce leaves (about 6 leaves)
½ cup (about 2 ounces) green pea sprouts
2 tablespoons tahini
¼ teaspoon sea salt
5 ounces (about 1 cup) frozen pineapple chunks
Handful of ice cubes

In a high-speed blender, combine all the ingredients in the order listed and blend, starting on low speed and working your way up to high, until smooth, about 2 minutes. Add more water if the smoothie is too thick. Pour into a glass and enjoy immediately.

> **TIP:** *Add liquid ingredients to your smoothies first; this will help get the blender going so the sprouts fully break down and blend in easily. But a stray unblended sprout will add textural interest to your smoothie!*

AVOCADO SALAD SMOOTHIE

Avocado pairs with cooling cucumber, mung, and lentil sprouts
to fuel your morning or swoop you out of that midday slump.
It's creamy, savory, and light yet substantial. To add a hint of
sweetness, swap coconut water for the plain water.

Serves 1

> ¾ cup water
> 1 medium cucumber (about 8 ounces), including peel
>   and seeds, chopped
> 2 tablespoons fresh lime juice
> ½ ripe avocado, chopped
> 2 cups (about 4 ounces) mature mung bean sprouts
> ¼ cup (about 1 ounce) lentil sprouts
> ¼ teaspoon sea salt
> Handful of ice cubes

In a high-speed blender, combine all the ingredients in the
order listed and blend, starting on low speed and working
your way up to high, until smooth, about 2 minutes. Add
more water if the smoothie is too thick. Pour into a glass and
enjoy immediately.

GINGER BROCCOLI SPROUT SMOOTHIE

You can't beat a hefty serving of one of the world's healthi-est foods—broccoli sprouts, with their mega-cancer-fighting sulforaphane—for the base of your smoothie. What a way to get serious about this superfood!

Serves 1

> 1 cup unsweetened almond milk, preferably Sprouted
> Almond Milk (page 169)
> 1 cup (about 1 ounce) broccoli sprouts
> 1 cup chopped fresh cilantro leaves and stems
> 1 medium cucumber (about 8 ounces), including peel
> and seeds, chopped
> ½ ripe avocado, chopped
> ½ lemon, peeled
> 2 teaspoons finely chopped ginger
> ¼ teaspoon sea salt
> Handful of ice cubes

In a high-speed blender, combine all the ingredients in the order listed and blend, starting on low speed and working your way up to high, until smooth, about 2 minutes. Add a little water or more almond milk if the smoothie is too thick. Pour into a glass and enjoy immediately.

CREAMY CACAO SMOOTHIE

For those who like their smoothies slightly sweet but still boasting superfood status. Feel free to swap another seasonal berry, such as blueberries or blackberries, for the raspberries.

Serves 1

 ½ cup unsweetened almond milk, preferably Sprouted
  Almond Milk (page 169)
 ¼ cup (about 1 ounce) green pea sprouts
 ½ cup (about ½ ounce) broccoli sprouts or other mild
  salad sprout
 1 dried Medjool date, pitted
 ¼ cup frozen raspberries
 ½ frozen banana
 1½ tablespoons raw cacao powder
 ⅛ teaspoon ground cinnamon
 Dash of almond extract (optional)
 Pinch of sea salt
 1 teaspoon fresh lemon juice, or to taste
 Handful of ice cubes

In a high-speed blender, combine all the ingredients in the order listed and blend, starting on low speed and working your way up to high, until smooth, about 2 minutes. Add a little water or more almond milk if the smoothie is too thick. Pour into a glass and enjoy immediately.

FROSTY ORANGE SMOOTHIE

This take on the classic Julius is a playful way to get a serious amount of sprouts into your system in one shot. And unlike the original, it will give you a protein boost rather than put you into sugar shock. Make sure to use mature mung bean sprouts that are more sprout than bean for this.

Serves 2 to 3

> 3 large oranges, peeled and segmented
> ½ cup (120 ml) unsweetened almond milk, preferably
>   Sprouted Almond Milk (page 169)
> 4 dried Medjool dates, pitted and chopped
> 1 teaspoon pure vanilla powder or extract
> ⅛ teaspoon ground turmeric
> 4 cups (about 8 ounces) mature mung bean sprouts
> ½ cup (about ½ ounce) mild vegetable sprout, such as
>   clover or alfalfa
> 1 small carrot, chopped
> Large handful of ice cubes

In a high-speed blender, combine all the ingredients in the order listed and blend, starting on low speed and working your way up to high, until smooth, about 2 minutes. Add a little water or more almond milk if the drink is too thick. Pour into glasses and enjoy immediately. Store leftovers in a tightly sealed jar for up to 1 day. Shake well before serving.

LEMON-LIME ELECTROLYTE DRINK

Ditch those sketchy colored waters you find at the supermarket. You don't need a bottleful of sugar to quench your thirst or fuel your workouts. Mung bean sprouts act like liquid and add protein, bonus vitamins A and C, and fiber to take hydration to a totally new level. The recipe contains a very generous four ounces of mung bean sprouts per serving. Healthiest quarter pounder ever! For a hint of sweetness, swap in coconut water for the plain water. Feel free to use all lemon or all lime juice if that's what you've got. Make sure to use mature mung bean sprouts that are more sprout than bean for this.

Serves 2

> 1 cup water
> 1 tablespoon fresh lime juice
> 1 tablespoon fresh lemon juice
> 2 whole sprigs mint, including stems (about ½ ounce), chopped
> 4 cups (about 8 ounces) mature mung bean sprouts
> ¼ teaspoon sea salt
> Handful of ice cubes

In a high-speed blender, combine all the ingredients in the order listed and blend, starting on low speed and working your way up to high, until smooth, about 2 minutes. Pour into glasses and enjoy immediately.

APPLE-CINNAMON OATMEAL

A bowl of oatmeal can be a comforting breakfast food, but it can also leave us with a bellyache. Before you give up oatmeal or any other grain, try soaking and sprouting that grain to remove difficult-to-digest antinutrients. It just might do the trick! Seasoning the oatmeal with fall spices and warming it slightly adds a comfort food effect while retaining the live enzymes of the grain.

Serves 2

>   2 cups (about 6 ounces) sprouted oats
>   1 cup unsweetened almond milk, preferably Sprouted
>   Almond Milk (page 169), plus more as needed
>   1 large apple, cored and chopped
>   ¼ cup raisins or currants
>   ½ teaspoon ground cinnamon, plus more for topping
>   ⅛ teaspoon ground nutmeg
>   ¼ teaspoon vanilla powder or extract
>   ⅛ teaspoon sea salt
>   ¼ cup chopped pecans or walnuts

In a small food processor or blender, combine the oats, almond milk, apple, raisins, cinnamon, nutmeg, vanilla powder, and salt and process until the oats and apples are broken down to a chunky mixture. Place in a small pot and heat until just warm but not hot. Spoon into bowls, top with the pecans and a little cinnamon, and serve.

CREAMY BUCKWHEAT CEREAL

Naturally gluten-free buckwheat grows a diminutive tail when sprouted, making it completely edible in its raw state. Buckwheat is high in protein and helps stabilize blood sugar, making it a smart choice for breakfast. Serve it at room temperature, or gently warm the almond milk to take off the chill. If you have a food dehydrator, you can warm it slightly in there.

Serves 4

    4 dried Medjool dates, pitted
    2 cups (about 8 ounces) sprouted buckwheat, divided
    ½ cup unsweetened almond milk, preferably Sprouted
       Almond Milk (page 169), plus more for serving
    ½ teaspoon ground cinnamon
    ½ teaspoon pure vanilla powder or extract
    Pinch of sea salt
    Topping options: fresh berries, sliced banana, almond
    slivers, coconut flakes, dried goji berries, a dusting of
    nutmeg, cacao nibs

1. Place the dates in a small bowl and add hot (not boiling) water to cover. Leave to soften for 20 minutes. Drain, reserving the soaking liquid.
2. In a food processor, combine the dates, 1½ cups of the sprouted buckwheat, the almond milk, cinnamon, vanilla, and salt and process until smooth. Add the remaining ½ cup buckwheat and pulse to combine (to give your porridge some texture).

If the mixture is too thick, pulse in some of the date-soaking water to reach your desired consistency. Spoon into bowls and serve with a drizzle of almond milk and your choice of toppings.

SOUPS AND SPREADS

MINTY GREEN PEA GAZPACHO

This soup is light, refreshing, and potent; sip up and feel the energy flow directly into your body! To serve your soup warm rather than chilled, blend it a little longer, until it's slightly heated (but not steaming hot, or it will lose its live enzymes). As long as your cucumber is organic, no need to peel or seed it; the peel adds to the vibrant green color of the soup, and your high-speed blender will break both the peel and seeds down to smooth submission. For a creamy garnish, top with a spoonful of Cashew Cream (page 208), or to simplify, pour into a glass, skip the garnishes, and bottoms up!

Serves 4

½ cup water

1 large cucumber (about 12 ounces), chopped

3 cups (about 6 ounces) mature mung bean sprouts

2 teaspoons lemon zest

½ cup fresh lemon juice, or to taste

2 scallions, white, green parts, and roots, chopped

1 cup (about 4 ounces) green pea sprouts, plus more for garnish

1 bunch fresh mint, including stems, chopped

¼ cup chopped fresh parsley leaves and stems

1¼ teaspoons sea salt, or to taste

⅛ teaspoon cayenne pepper, or to taste

¼ cup extra-virgin olive oil, plus more for drizzling

Garnish options: Pea shoots or sunflower shoots, scallions, paprika

In a high-speed blender, combine the water, cucumber, mung bean sprouts, lemon zest, lemon juice, scallions, pea sprouts, mint, parsley, salt, and cayenne in that order and blend, starting on low speed and working your way up to high, until silky smooth, 3 to 4 minutes, adding more water if the soup is too thick. Lower the speed to medium and add the oil through the hole in the lid; blend until incorporated. Taste and add more salt and/or lemon juice if needed. Serve immediately, or transfer to a container and refrigerate until cold, at least 2 hours or overnight. Taste the soup again and adjust the seasonings if needed. Divide the soup into bowls, finish with a drizzle of oil and a sprinkle of sprouted peas, and serve.

Variation: CILANTRO-LIME GREEN PEA GAZPACHO
Swap ¼ cup fresh lime juice for the lemon juice and 2 cups chopped fresh cilantro leaves and stems for the mint and parsley.

TOMATO AND ONION SPROUT SOUP

Onion sprouts, with their tiny black seed heads, are stunning to look at and impart a powerfully pungent flavor to this simple blender soup. The soup gets its creaminess from cashews, and mung bean sprouts provide a liquid base. Make sure to use mature mung bean sprouts that are more sprout than bean for this. To serve the soup warm, let the blender go for a few more minutes.

Serves 4 (makes about 5 cups)

> ½ cup raw cashews
> ¼ cup sun-dried tomatoes (not oil-packed)
> 1½ pounds fresh tomatoes (4 large), chopped
> 1¼ cups water
> 1 cup (about 2 ounces) mature mung bean sprouts
> 1 cup (about 1 ounce) onion sprouts, plus more for garnish
> 1 garlic clove, peeled
> 1½ tablespoons fresh lime juice, or to taste
> 1 teaspoon sea salt, or to taste
> ¾ teaspoon paprika
> ½ teaspoon garlic powder
> ½ cup (½ ounce) packed fresh Thai or Italian basil leaves

1. Place the cashews in a small bowl and add hot (not boiling) water to cover. Place the sun-dried tomatoes in a separate bowl and add hot (not boiling) water to cover. Leave the

cashews and sun-dried tomatoes to soak until softened, about 2 hours. Drain.

2. In a high-speed blender, combine the fresh tomatoes, water, mung bean sprouts, onion sprouts, garlic, lime juice, salt, paprika, and garlic powder in that order and blend, starting on low speed and working your way up to high, until silky smooth, 3 to 4 minutes, adding more water if the soup is too thick. If the blender starts to get hot, stop to cool it for a couple of minutes. Taste and add more salt or lime juice if needed. Add the basil and pulse until combined. Serve immediately, or transfer to a container and refrigerate until cold, at least 2 hours or overnight. Taste the soup again and adjust the seasonings if needed. Divide the soup into bowls or cups, finish with a handful of onion sprouts, and serve.

NEW CLASSIC HUMMUS

Alive with sprouted chickpeas and zucchini for added veggie goodness, this will forever change your conception of hummus. Roll some into a veggie wrap or grab a carrot stick and have at it!

Makes about 3 cups

¼ cup fresh lemon juice, or to taste

2 garlic cloves, chopped

1 cup (about 2 ounces) mature mung bean sprouts

1 medium zucchini (about 6 ounces), including stem, chopped

½ cup tahini

1 cup (about 4 ounces) chickpea sprouts

½ teaspoon ground cumin

1 teaspoon sea salt, or to taste

½ teaspoon freshly ground black pepper, or to taste

¼ cup extra-virgin olive oil, plus more for drizzling

2 tablespoons chopped fresh parsley

Sprinkle of paprika

In a high-speed blender, combine the lemon juice, garlic, mung bean sprouts, zucchini, tahini, chickpea sprouts, cumin, salt, and pepper in that order and blend, starting on low speed and working your way up to high, until silky smooth, 3 to 4 minutes, scraping down the sides as needed and adding water if the mixture is too thick. If the blender starts to get hot, stop to cool it for a couple of minutes. Add the oil and blend on low speed for about 30 seconds, until well combined. Add the parsley and pulse it in. Taste and add more lemon juice, salt, and/or pepper as needed. Transfer to a bowl or container and, if you have time, let sit for about 30 minutes to allow the flavors to blend, then taste again and adjust the seasonings as needed. Serve topped with a drizzle of oil and a sprinkle of paprika. The hummus will keep, covered tightly, for up to 5 days in the refrigerator.

ALKALIZING LEMON WATER

After squeezing your lemons for juice, save the rinds and add
them to a pitcher of water. Leave to soak for 30 minutes to
1 hour, then remove them (longer than that and the water
will become overly astringent) and sip on the alkalizing lemon
water throughout the day to set your system straight (or keep
it that way).

MUSHROOM-LENTIL PÂTÉ

Rich, smooth, and a little sweet, this pâté punctuated with porcinis delivers a serious hit of umami. It's the baddest dip to hit a veggie stick since hummus (see the new classic version on pages 183–184), and spread over thick cucumber slices, it becomes an unforgettable passed app. To make a meal of it, stuff it into a collard leaf wrap (page 197).

Makes about 3 cups

½ cup dried porcini mushrooms

1 cup hot (not boiling) water

1 cup (about 4 ounces) lentil sprouts

1 cup (about 2 ounces) mature mung bean sprouts

1 cup raw walnut halves

½ cup olive oil–packed sun-dried tomatoes, chopped

2 tablespoons coconut aminos

1½ tablespoons raw apple cider vinegar, or to taste

1 teaspoon dried marjoram

1 teaspoon dried thyme

1 teaspoon garlic powder

1 teaspoon onion powder

¼ teaspoon freshly ground black pepper

¼ teaspoon cayenne pepper

¼ teaspoon ground cumin

½ teaspoon sea salt, or to taste

¼ cup extra-virgin olive oil

Optional garnishes: chopped fresh parsley, snipped chives, a sprinkle of paprika, extra lentil sprouts, extra

minced sun-dried tomatoes, sliced raw pickles, pickled
red onions (pages 197–198)

Put the mushrooms in a small bowl and pour the hot water
over them. Leave to soak for 1 to 2 hours, until softened.
Remove the hydrated mushrooms from the water and put
them in a high-speed blender. Put a mesh strainer over the
blender and line it with a coffee filter or paper towel. Strain
the soaking liquid through the filter directly into the blender.
Add the lentil sprouts, mung bean sprouts, walnuts, sun-dried
tomatoes, coconut aminos, vinegar, marjoram, thyme, garlic
powder, onion powder, black pepper, cayenne, cumin, and
salt and blend, starting on low speed and working your way
up to high, until very smooth, about 5 minutes, stopping to
prevent the mixture from getting too warm and to scrape
the sides of the machine as needed. Add the oil and blend
until incorporated. Taste and add more vinegar and/or salt if
needed. The pâté will keep, covered in the refrigerator, for up
to 5 days.

TIP: *Swap deeply detoxifying shiitakes or another dried
mushroom to change up the flavor and nutritional profile of
your pâté.*

KIM CHEESE DIP

Daikon sprouts add a pungent radish bite to kimchi's fiery heat, and cashews provide a creamy base to this vegan cheese dip. To tone it down, swap in a non-spicy sprout, such as alfalfa or clover, or scoop the dip up with sticks of cooling mature daikon.

Makes about 1½ cups

> 1 cup raw cashews
> 1 cup vegan kimchi, drained
> 1 cup (about 1 ounce) daikon radish sprouts

1. Place the cashews in a small bowl and add hot (not boiling) water to cover. Leave to soak until softened, about 2 hours. Drain.
2. Combine all the ingredients in a food processor and process to a coarse puree. Scrape into a bowl and serve with vegetable sticks for dipping. The dip will keep, covered and refrigerated, for up to 1 week.

CRUNCHY CHICKPEA CHAAT WITH TWO CHUTNEYS AND CASHEW CREAM

This clean, energizing version of a popular Indian street food will not only get you closer to your health goals, it doubles as party food! Make a big batch, set up bowls of each ingredient, and invite your guests to mix and match to make their own chaat. Chaat masala is a spice mix with a unique sulfury flavor that is quite addictive. You'll find it in Indian grocery stores.

Serves 4

4 cups (about 1 pound) chickpea sprouts, divided
1 small red onion or 4 scallions, white and green parts, chopped
1 large tomato, chopped
1 small cucumber, chopped
1 cup Cilantro-Mint Chutney (pages 214–215)
½ cup Tamarind Chutney (recipe follows)
½ cup Cashew Cream (page 208)
4 large pinches of chaat masala
2 pinches of ground cumin
4 pinches of mild chile powder (optional)

4 pinches of flaky sea salt
Mature mung bean sprouts, for topping

In a large bowl, combine the chickpea sprouts, onion, tomato, and cucumber. Divide the mixture among four bowls. Pour the chutneys and cashew cream onto each bowl and top with the chaat masala, cumin, chile powder, if using, salt, and mung bean sprouts. Serve immediately, instructing diners to mix everything up on the spot.

TIP: *To simplify, omit the Tamarind Chutney and/or Cashew Cream.*

TAMARIND CHUTNEY
Makes about ½ cup

⅓ cup tamarind puree (see Note)
¼ cup packed dried, pitted Medjool dates
2 tablespoons water, or as needed
Pinch of ground cumin
Pinch of sea salt

In a mini blender or food processor, combine all the ingredients and blend until smooth. The chutney will keep, covered and refrigerated, for up to 2 weeks.

Note: *Make sure to use tamarind puree, not the thick, dark concentrate paste.*

SPROUTS AND KRAUT

Sprouts and kraut are two of the most potent living foods you can eat. When you combine them, you experience mega-nutrition and a tangy, crunchy taste experience. Add oil to the juice from the kraut and you have an instant salad dressing. Onion sprouts add a pungent, spicy finish to this super salad; for milder tastes, swap in clover sprouts or another mild leafy green sprout.

Serves 1 to 2

- 1 cup raw sauerkraut, plus additional juice from the jar
- 1 cup (about 4 ounces) green pea sprouts or other crunchy sprout
- 1 cup (about 1 ounce) broccoli sprouts
- 1 small cucumber, cubed
- ½ cup dulse fronds
- 1½ tablespoons extra-virgin olive oil
- ¼ cup (about ¼ ounce) onion sprouts
- 1 tablespoon raw pumpkin seeds
- 1 tablespoon sunflower seeds, preferably sprouted

In a salad bowl, combine the sauerkraut, pea sprouts, broccoli sprouts, cucumber, and dulse and toss to coat and soften the dulse. Add the oil and toss to coat. Taste and add juice from the sauerkraut jar until the salad is tangy to your liking. Top with the onion sprouts, pumpkin seeds, and sunflower seeds and serve.

> **TIP:** *Try a flavored sauerkraut, such as caraway or turmeric, or swap in vegan kimchi for the kraut.*

JEAN-GEORGES'S CARROT AND AVOCADO SALAD

This salad comes courtesy of Michelin-starred chef Jean-Georges Vongerichten. While there's a cooked element to it (the rest of the recipes in the book are fully raw), this recipe makes it clear that sprouts are making their way into the world's finest kitchens!

Serves 4

> 1 pound medium carrots
>
> 3 garlic cloves, peeled
>
> 1 teaspoon cumin seeds
>
> 1 teaspoon fresh thyme leaves
>
> ¼ teaspoon red chile flakes
>
> Sea salt and freshly ground black pepper
>
> 1 tablespoon red wine vinegar
>
> ¼ cup plus 2 tablespoons extra-virgin olive oil
>
> 1½ oranges
>
> 2 lemons, cut in half
>
> 1 tablespoon sunflower seeds
>
> 1 tablespoon pumpkin seeds
>
> 1 tablespoon white sesame seeds
>
> 1 avocado, cut into thin wedges
>
> 4 cups sprouts, preferably a mix of radish and beet

1. Preheat the oven to 350°F.
2. Bring a wide pot of water to a boil. Add the carrots and cook until a knife pierces them easily, about 20 minutes.

3. Meanwhile, in a mortar and pestle, pound the garlic, cumin, thyme, chile flakes, 1½ teaspoons salt, and ¾ teaspoon pepper until crushed and pasty. Add the vinegar and ¼ cup of the oil and continue pounding until well mixed. Alternatively, pulse in a food processor or blender until pasty.

4. Drain the carrots and arrange them in a medium roasting pan in a single layer. Spoon the cumin mixture over them. Cut the whole orange in half. Arrange the orange halves and 2 of the lemon halves over the carrots, cut-side down. Roast for 25 minutes, or until the carrots are golden brown. Transfer the carrots to a platter.

5. While the carrots are in the oven, spread the sunflower, pumpkin, and sesame seeds on a baking sheet in a single layer. Toast, stirring occasionally, until golden but not golden brown, about 7 minutes. Remove from the oven and cool completely.

6. When cool enough to handle, squeeze 2 tablespoons juice each from the roasted orange and lemon into a small bowl. Squeeze in 2 tablespoons orange juice from the remaining orange half and 2 tablespoons lemon juice from the remaining lemon. Whisk in the remaining 2 tablespoons oil to emulsify. Season with salt and pepper and drizzle over the carrots.

7. Arrange the carrots on a serving platter, reserving the accompanying sauce. Top with the avocado and sprouts. Drizzle with the reserved sauce and sprinkle with the seeds. Serve immediately.

MADKI (INDIAN RAW SPROUT SALAD)

In India, a country with its fair share of vegetarians, sprouts are a fantastic source of affordable protein. This sprout salad, spiced with red onion, chile, and a salty, sulfury spice mix known as *chaat masala* is a superfood you can really get excited about. You also could make your madki with young mung bean sprouts, which are mostly beans with little tails (not the fully sprouted mung beans you typically see in Asian stir-fries and other dishes).

Serves 1

2 cups (about 4 ounces) adzuki bean sprouts

1 medium tomato, chopped

½ small red onion, chopped

½ to 1 fresh green chile, thinly sliced

2 tablespoons chopped almonds

2 teaspoons fresh lime juice, or to taste

½ teaspoon chaat masala, plus more for sprinkling

¼ teaspoon sea salt, or to taste

1 ripe avocado, sliced

In a salad bowl, combine the sprouts, tomato, red onion, green chile, almonds, lime juice, chaat masala, and salt. Top with the avocado and a sprinkle of chaat masala and serve.

ZUCCHINI NOODLES AND SPROUTS WITH SPICY GINGER-LIME ALMOND DRESSING

This healthy take on pasta just got twenty times healthier—and more delicious—by adding sprouts to the mix! The sauce doubles as a dip for vegetable sticks or can be tossed with another salad with sturdy greens and sprouts.

Serves 2

Spicy Ginger-Lime Almond Dressing

½ cup smooth almond butter

¼ cup warm water, or as needed

3 tablespoons coconut aminos

1 teaspoon dulse granules

3 tablespoons fresh lime juice, or to taste

1 teaspoon grated fresh ginger

½ teaspoon cayenne pepper

½ teaspoon sea salt

1 garlic clove, pressed through a garlic press

Salad

2 cups zucchini noodles

2 cups (about 4 ounces) mature mung bean sprouts

2 cups (about 3 ounces) sunflower shoots or pea shoots

1 small carrot, grated or spiralized

1 small red bell pepper, thinly sliced

1 small tomato, chopped

2 scallions, white and green parts, sliced

¼ cup chopped fresh flat-leaf parsley

¼ cup chopped fresh mint

½ teaspoon sea salt

2 tablespoons slivered almonds, preferably sprouted

1. To make the dressing: In a medium bowl, whisk together all the ingredients until smooth. Add more water if it's too thick and more lime juice if needed.

2. To make the salad: Combine all the ingredients in a large bowl. Add half the dressing and toss to coat. Spoon into bowls and serve. The remaining dressing will keep, covered, for up to 1 week.

MUSHROOM-LENTIL PÂTÉ AND PICKLED SPROUT WRAPS

Mushroom-forward flavor with pickled sprouts adding crunchy bursts of tang make this a wrap to remember. This dish will make anyone a sprout believer!

Makes 2 wraps

>2 collard leaves
>1 cup Mushroom-Lentil Pâté (pages 186–187)
>1 cup (about 1 ounce) broccoli, radish, clover, or alfalfa sprouts, or a mix
>1 small tomato, chopped
>2 tablespoons Quick Pickled Sprouts (recipe follows), plus a little pickling liquid

1. Freeze the collard leaves for 10 minutes (this makes it easier to trim the stems). Trim the stems from the bottom and outer part of the leaves to make the leaves bendable.

2. Spread the pâté over the collard leaves and top with the sprouts, tomato, and pickled sprouts and roll them up. Trim the edges (and eat them) and cut in half if you like. Place on a plate seam side down and serve immediately.

QUICK PICKLED SPROUTS

For a lively zing of flavor, add to wraps, salads, or soups, and be sure to include a splash of vinegar. Use any firm, crunchy sprouts, such as mung, chickpea, lentil, or pea.
Makes as much as you like

Sprouts or onion slices
Raw apple cider vinegar

Put the sprouts or onion in a jar. Add vinegar to cover. Leave to pickle for 15 minutes, strain (and save the vinegar to use in a dressing), then use immediately.

GREEN PEA AVOCADO CREAM AND CHIA SPROUT WRAPS

Creamy, crunchy, and filled with omega-3 fatty acids in easily accessible form from the sprouted chia, this wrap is a nutritional flavor force to be reckoned with! You could swap any sprout for the chia, and instead of carrot, you might try beet or shredded cabbage. Mix and match with what you have growing to showcase your sprout bounty.

Serves 2

> 2 collard leaves
> 1 cup Green Pea Avocado Cream (page 217)
> 1 cup (about 1 ounce) chia sprouts or sunflower or pea shoots
> 1 medium carrot, grated
> ½ lemon
> Flaky sea salt and freshly ground black pepper

1. Freeze the collard leaves for 10 minutes (this makes it easier to trim the stems). Trim the stems from the bottom and outer part of the leaves to make the leaves bendable.
2. Spread the avocado cream over the collard leaves and top with the chia sprouts and carrot. Finish with a squeeze of lemon and a pinch of salt and pepper and roll them up. Trim the edges (and eat them) and cut in half if you like. Place on a plate seam side down and serve immediately.

LEMONY CAULIFLOWER SALAD

Lots of cleansing lemon kisses detoxifying, cancer-fighting cauliflower in this cruciferous salad punctuated by a mix of crunchy, proteinaceous sprouts. Use any crunchy sprout mix, such as a combination of green peas, lentils, and adzuki beans, or a single sprout if that's what's available. This salad makes use of all the cauliflower—florets, stems, core, and leaves—so nothing goes to waste. Preserved lemon can be found in specialty stores or online. Rinse them of extra salt before using. If unavailable, substitute the zest of 2 lemons.

Serves 4

¼ cup currants

1 small head (about 1½ pounds) cauliflower

2 cups (about 8 ounces) mixed crunchy sprouts

½ preserved lemon, finely chopped

½ cup chopped almonds, preferably sprouted

¼ cup fresh lemon juice

1 teaspoon sea salt

¼ teaspoon cayenne pepper

3 tablespoons extra-virgin olive oil

¼ cup chopped fresh flat-leaf parsley

¼ cup chopped fresh mint

¼ cup (about ¼ ounce) fenugreek sprouts (optional)

1. Soak the currants in hot (not boiling) water to cover for about 15 minutes while you prep your ingredients.

2. Trim the cauliflower of its leaves and finely chop the leaves; set aside. Cut the cauliflower into approximately 1-inch pieces (include the stems), then, working in two batches, pulse until broken down into pieces between the size of chickpeas and rice (it's fine if the texture isn't even). Place in a bowl along with the leaves and add the currants, sprout mix, preserved lemon, and sprouted almonds.

3. In a small bowl, whisk together the lemon juice, salt, and cayenne, then slowly whisk in the oil until emulsified. Add to the cauliflower mixture and toss to fully coat. Add the parsley and mint. If you have the time, leave the salad on the counter for up to 1 hour to marinate, then spoon into bowls, top with the fenugreek sprouts, if using, and serve.

QUINOA TABBOULEH

Swapping out the wheat for quinoa and sprouting it brings new life to this classic grain-based salad. It's best enjoyed at the height of tomato season. Depending on your tomatoes, the tabbouleh can get pretty juicy after it's all mixed. If it looks overly moist, drain it slightly and use the flavorful liquid to toss into a future bowl of sprouts.

Serves 4

  2 cups sprouted quinoa, patted dry with a paper towel
    if damp
  2 large tomatoes, seeded and diced
  3 tablespoons fresh lemon juice, or to taste, divided
  ½ teaspoon ground coriander
  ½ teaspoon sea salt, divided
  1 large cucumber, seeded and chopped
  1 cup chopped fresh flat-leaf parsley
  ½ cup chopped fresh mint
  2 scallions, white and green parts, thinly sliced
  ½ teaspoon freshly ground black pepper
  3 tablespoons extra-virgin olive oil
  Romaine lettuce leaves or your choice of sprout for
    serving
  ½ cup (about ½ ounce) fenugreek sprouts (optional)

In a large bowl, combine the sprouted quinoa, tomatoes, 2 tablespoons of the lemon juice, the coriander, and ¼ teaspoon of the salt. Let stand for 30 minutes, then add the cucumber, parsley, mint, and scallions. Add the remaining ¼ teaspoon salt, the pepper, the remaining 1 tablespoon lemon juice, and the oil. Serve over lettuce leaves and top with the fenugreek sprouts, if using.

HOUSE SPROUT SALAD

This everyday go-to salad can be changed up according to season, whim, or what's in your fridge or growing in your sprout garden at any time. You can swap in any type of crunchy sprout and veggie, keeping a more or less 1:1 ratio of sprouts to veggies. Double or triple the dressing for sprout salad making throughout the week. Because all the components of the salad are sturdy, leftover dressed salad can be kept refrigerated overnight.

Serves 2 to 4

Dressing

2 tablespoons fresh lime juice

1 clove garlic, pressed through a garlic press

¼ teaspoon flaky sea salt

2 teaspoons minced fresh rosemary, thyme, oregano, or
  a mix

¼ teaspoon freshly ground black pepper

¼ cup extra-virgin olive oil

Salad

3 cups (about 12 ounces) mixed crunchy sprouts, such
  as green pea, chickpea, and adzuki bean

1 small cucumber, chopped

1 large carrot, chopped

1 large celery stalk, chopped

1 cup mixed fresh soft herbs, such as cilantro, parsley,
  and chives

Sea salt and freshly ground black pepper to taste

Optional add-ins: sliced avocado, chopped nuts, sesame or poppy seeds, sauerkraut, olives, capers, ripped nori sheet

1. To make the dressing: Pour the lime juice into a small bowl. Add the garlic, salt, herbs, and pepper, then whisk in the oil until emulsified. (Alternatively, combine all the ingredients in a jar, cover, and shake until emulsified.)
2. To put together the salad: In a large bowl, combine all the salad ingredients and toss. Add the dressing (you may have some left over), toss to coat, and serve.

AVOCADO SPROUT BOATS WITH CLOVER CHERMOULA

An avocado boat makes a playful platform for any sprout salad. If you haven't made the chermoula, try using Pumped-Up Pesto (pages 219–220) or toss your sprouts with House Sprout Salad dressing (page 204) or a simple mix of olive oil and lemon juice.

Serves 2 as a starter or snack

> 1 large ripe avocado
> ¼ cup Clover Chermoula (page 218)
> ½ cup (about ½ ounce) clover sprouts or other sprouts of your choice

Cut the avocado in half and remove the pit. Spoon 1 tablespoon chermoula over each avocado half, top with the sprouts, and finish with the remaining chermoula. Serve immediately.

TIP: *Avocado boats also welcome New Classic Hummus (pages 184–185), Mushroom-Lentil Pâté (pages 186–187), or Kim Cheese Dip (page 188).*

GARAM MASALA LENTILS, CAULIFLOWER RICE, ORANGE, AND CASHEW CREAM

Cauliflower and crunchy sprouts get a toss with warming spices and cheerful citrus, and a dollop of cashew cream pulls the dish together. Revelation: Cauliflower leaves are every bit as nutritious and tasty as the florets. Don't leave them out! You can swap adzuki bean sprouts or sprouted green peas for the lentil sprouts.

Serves 2

2 cups Cauliflower Rice (recipe follows)
1 cup (about 4 ounces) lentil sprouts or any mix of
   crunchy sprouts
1 large orange
2 teaspoons fresh lime juice
½ teaspoon garam masala
¼ teaspoon ground fennel
¼ teaspoon cumin seeds
¼ teaspoon salt
¼ teaspoon freshly ground black pepper
1 tablespoon extra-virgin olive oil
Cashew Cream (recipe follows)
Julienned cauliflower leaves, for garnish

1. In a large bowl, combine the cauliflower rice and lentil sprouts.
2. Zest the orange, then cut the orange in half. Peel and chop half of the orange and juice the other half into a small bowl.

Add the lime juice, most of the orange zest (reserve a pinch for garnish), the garam masala, fennel, cumin seeds, salt, and pepper, and whisk to dissolve the seasonings. Whisk in the oil.

3. Pour the dressing over the cauliflower and lentil sprouts and mix to combine and fully coat the ingredients. Divide into bowls, top each with a dollop of cashew cream, a sprinkle of orange zest, and some cauliflower leaves, and serve.

CASHEW CREAM
Makes about 1 cup

1 cup raw unsalted cashews
Pinch of sea salt

1. Place the cashews in a medium bowl and add hot (not boiling) water to cover by a couple of inches. Set aside for at least 2 hours or up to overnight. Drain.

2. Transfer the cashews to a blender (a mini blender works great for this), add ⅓ cup water and the salt, and blend, starting on low speed and working your way up to high, until smooth, about 3 minutes, stopping to scrape the sides as needed. Use immediately or transfer to an airtight container and refrigerate for up to 1 week.

CAULIFLOWER RICE
Makes about 8 cups

1 (3-pound) head cauliflower

1. Quarter the cauliflower through the core, then cut out the core and leaves from each quarter in one cut. Remove any remaining core and leaves.

2. Break the cauliflower into 2-inch florets. Put half of the cauliflower in a food processor and pulse about 20 times, until the florets are about the size of rice, scraping the sides of the machine once or twice if needed. Remove from the machine to a bowl and repeat with the remaining cauliflower. Use immediately, or cover and refrigerate for up to 3 days.

CRUNCHY SPROUT, CELERY, AND APPLE SALAD WITH GOLDEN TAHINI DRESSING

This light yet satisfying salad is all about the crunch. Tahini dressing adds a creamy counterpoint, and pomegranate seeds give it a hit of ruby bliss. If you haven't sprouted sesame seeds for the tahini dressing, it's fine to use un-sprouted sesame seeds. You'll still be getting a generous serving of sprouts in your salad.

Serves 2

> 1 cup (about 4 ounces) lentil or other crunchy sprouts
> 3 stalks celery, thinly sliced
> 1 small apple, cored and chopped
> ¼ cup Golden Tahini Dressing (page 216), plus more
>   for drizzling
> 2 to 3 tablespoons pomegranate seeds
> Celery leaves, for garnish
> Fenugreek sprouts (optional), for garnish

In a serving bowl, combine the sprouts, celery, and apple. Add the dressing and toss to coat. Top with a drizzle of dressing, follow by the pomegranate seeds, celery leaves, and fenugreek sprouts, if using, and serve.

UNFRIED KIMCHI RICE AND ADZUKI SPROUT BOWL

Get your spice on with this sprout-full take on the Korean classic. Look for sugar-free, vegan kimchi to keep the dish plant-based and choose a brand with no added sugar. Coconut aminos are a gluten-free, soy-free substitute for soy sauce; adjust the amount depending on how salty your kimchi is.

2 cups Cauliflower Rice (see pages 208–209)

1 cup vegan kimchi, plus kimchi juice if needed

1 cup (about 4 ounces) adzuki bean sprouts or other crunchy sprout

1 tablespoon coconut aminos, or to taste

2 teaspoons toasted sesame oil

1 avocado, sliced or chopped

1 sheet nori, cut into thin strips

1 scallion, white and green parts, thinly sliced on a diagonal

2 teaspoons black sesame seeds

In a medium bowl, combine the cauliflower, kimchi, and sprouts. Add the coconut aminos and sesame oil and stir to coat. Add some kimchi juice from the jar if it needs more juice. Spoon into bowls, place the avocado on one side, and top with the nori, scallion, and sesame seeds. Serve immediately.

JICAMA RICE AND BEANS WITH REALLY GREEN SALSA

Rice made from the root jicama is sweet and super crunchy, making it the perfect base for a sproutarian rice-and-beans bowl. To vary the recipe, you could sub 2 cups Cauliflower Rice for the jicama, and instead of the adzuki sprouts, you could use sprouted green peas or chickpeas.

Serves 2

> 1 small jicama (about 1½ pounds)
> 1 cup (about 4 ounces) adzuki bean sprouts
> 1 cup Really Green Salsa (page 221)
> Garnishes: sunflower sprouts (shoots), shredded carrot,
>   avocado slices, Quick Pickled Sprouts (pages 197–198)

1. Peel the jicama and cut it into ½-inch cubes. Place it in the food processor and pulse until it is broken down to a rice-like texture.
2. Transfer the jicama to a nut milk bag and squeeze to extract most of the liquid. If you don't have a nut milk bag, line a mesh strainer with a double layer of paper towel, add the jicama rice, and leave for 1 hour to drain. It will remove some of the liquid, but a nut milk bag will get you that al dente rice-like texture, making it worth the investment (especially because the nut milk bag can double as a sprouting bag).
3. Divide the jicama between two bowls and top with the sprouted adzuki beans and salsa. Finish with your choice of garnishes and serve.

CARROT AND DAIKON NOODLES WITH SUNFLOWER SHOOTS AND PUMPED-UP PESTO

Sweet carrots and juicy daikon radish stay crisp when spiralized and welcome a toss with a sprout-packed pesto. If you don't have a spiralizer, you could shred the carrots and daikon on the large holes of a box grater; you won't get the long, curly noodles a dedicated spiralizer produces, but the veggies will still be an efficient delivery system for the pesto. You also could swap in 3 cups store-bought zucchini noodles for the carrots and daikon.

Serves 2

> 2 large carrots
> 1 small daikon radish (about 8 ounces)
> ½ cup Pumped-Up Pesto (pages 219–220), plus more for
>   serving
> Sunflower or pea shoots, for garnish
> Pine nuts or other nuts, for garnish

Using a spiralizer, spiralize the carrots and radish into spaghetti shapes. Place in a large bowl, add the pesto, and toss to coat. Divide between two bowls or plates and top with sunflower shoots, additional pesto, and nuts, if using. Serve immediately.

SAUCES

CILANTRO-MINT CHUTNEY

Fresh, slightly grassy, and with a hint of spice, this chutney is a bold new addition to your sprout-forward kitchen. Thin it with olive oil to make a salad dressing, or finish a soup such as Minty Green Pea Gazpacho (pages 179–180) with a spoonful of it. You'll go crazy for it over chaat (pages 189–190).

Makes about 1½ cups

- ¼ cup water
- 2 tablespoons fresh lime juice
- 2 cups (about 4 ounces) mature mung bean sprouts
- 2 cups chopped fresh cilantro leaves and stems
- 2 cups chopped fresh mint leaves and stems
- ¼ cup raw cashew pieces
- 2 dried Medjool dates, pitted
- 2 teaspoons chopped fresh ginger
- 1 Indian green chile or jalapeño chile
- ¾ teaspoon sea salt, or to taste

In a small blender or mini food processor, combine all the ingredients in the order listed and blend until smooth, stopping to scrape the sides of the machine and adding more water if the chutney is too thick. This chutney is best served the day it's made but will keep covered and refrigerated overnight.

GOLDEN TAHINI DRESSING

Tahini is breaking out of the hummus-and-falafel box and making a splash in both savory and sweet dishes across cuisines. In this book, it's added to smoothies (page 170), halvah (pages 228–229), and this rich and creamy turmeric-tinted dressing. Tip: When you use turmeric, also use black pepper—they have a synergistic nutritional effect on each other.

Makes about 1 cup

> 1½ cups (about 5 ounces) sprouted sesame seeds
> ¾ cup water, or as needed
> 3 to 4 tablespoons fresh lemon juice, to taste
> 1 tablespoon extra-virgin olive oil
> ⅛ teaspoon ground turmeric
> ⅛ teaspoon freshly ground black pepper
> ¼ teaspoon sea salt

In a high-speed blender (a mini blender works well), combine all the ingredients and blend, starting on low speed and working your way up to high, until silky smooth, about 3 minutes. Store in an airtight container in the refrigerator for up to 3 days.

GREEN PEA AVOCADO CREAM

This is an avocado cream like no other. It's fortified by sprouted peas for protein, giving it a slightly grassy back note, and zucchini lightens it up a bit so you can eat more of it! Spread it into a collard leaf and pair it with a companion sprout to make a wrap (page 199), pull up some veggie sticks, or simply snack on a spoonful of it.

Makes about 1½ cups

> 1 large ripe avocado, chopped
> ½ cup (about 2 ounces) green pea sprouts
> 1 small zucchini (about 4 ounces), chopped
> 1 tablespoon fresh lime juice
> ½ teaspoon sea salt

In a high-speed blender, preferably a mini blender, combine all the ingredients and blend until smooth, about 3 minutes, scraping the sides once or twice as needed. Serve immediately, or store in a covered container in the refrigerator for up to 2 days.

CLOVER CHERMOULA

Chermoula is a potent sauce made with herbs, spices, garlic, and lemon juice. Sprouts aren't traditional, but they are hardly detected. You may use just about any salad green sprout, such as broccoli sprouts or alfalfa sprouts, or radish sprouts for a spicier chermoula.

Makes about 1½ cups

> 4 cloves garlic, peeled
> 2 cups (about 2 ounces) clover sprouts
> 1 cup packed chopped fresh cilantro leaves and stems
> 1 cup packed chopped fresh flat-leaf parsley leaves and stems
> 2 teaspoons grated lemon zest
> 2 teaspoons ground cumin
> 2 teaspoons paprika
> 1 teaspoon ground coriander
> 1 teaspoon sea salt
> 1 tablespoon fresh lime juice
> ½ cup extra-virgin olive oil

With the motor of a food processor running, drop the garlic through the hole in the lid to mince it. Scrape down the sides of the bowl. Add the sprouts, cilantro, parsley, lemon zest, cumin, paprika, coriander, salt, and lime juice and pulse to chop. With the motor running, drizzle the oil through the hole in the lid and process until broken down but with some texture remaining. Scrape into a jar, cover, and refrigerate until ready to use. It will keep for up to 3 days.

PUMPED-UP PESTO

If you are tiptoeing your way into sprouts, try adding sprouts to something you're already familiar with, like a pesto, by swapping the sprouts for part or all of the herb component. You won't notice they are there, which makes this even more of a game changer!

Makes about 1½ cups

- 1 garlic clove, peeled
- ½ cup pine nuts or pumpkin seeds
- 2 cups (about 2 ounces) broccoli sprouts or other salad green sprout
- 1 packed cup (about 1 ounce) fresh basil leaves and tender stems
- 1 packed cup (about 1 ounce) roughly chopped fresh cilantro leaves and tender stems
- ½ cup extra-virgin olive oil
- 1½ tablespoons fresh lemon juice, or to taste
- ¼ teaspoon sea salt, or to taste
- ¼ teaspoon freshly ground black pepper, or to taste
- Pinch of red pepper flakes (optional)

With the motor of a food processor running, drop the garlic through the hole in the lid to mince it. Stop the machine, add the pine nuts, and pulse until finely ground, about 1 minute. Add the broccoli sprouts, basil, cilantro, oil, lemon juice, salt, black pepper, and red pepper flakes, if using, and process until just about smooth, about 1 minute, stopping to scrape the sides of the machine as needed. Use immediately, or transfer to a jar, cover, and keep in the refrigerator for up to 2 days.

REALLY GREEN SALSA

Loads of cilantro and broccoli sprouts give this salsa an emerald-green color, and the seed heads from the broccoli sprouts show themselves off like precious jewels. This salsa is the essence of fresh!

Makes about 2 cups

> 1 pound tomatillos
> 2 cups roughly chopped fresh cilantro
> 1 small jalapeño chile, chopped
> 1 garlic clove, chopped
> 2 cups (about 2 ounces) broccoli sprouts or other salad sprouts
> ½ teaspoon sea salt

1. Remove the papery husks from the tomatillos and rinse them well.
2. In a food processor, combine all the ingredients and process to a salsa consistency. The salsa will keep covered in the refrigerator for up to 3 days.

SNACKS AND SWEETS

LIME AND CHILE SPROUTS

In the style of Mexican street fruit salad, a shower of lime, a sprinkle of salt, and a little chile powder transform a simple bowl of sprouts into a taste sensation. Choose any type of bean or vegetable sprout, such as pea, lentil, chickpea, broccoli, radish, clover, or a combination for variety in taste and texture. Maximum nutrition from minimal calories—enjoy often and abundantly!

Serves 1 to 2

    2 cups any type of sprout
    ½ lime
    Sprinkle of chile powder
    Sprinkle of flaky sea salt

Put the sprouts in a medium bowl. Squeeze on the lime and finish with the chile powder and salt. Serve immediately.

SPROUTS ON A LOG

A childhood classic snack transformed into a superfood! Choose any sprout you fancy, or a mix, to decorate your log and change up your nut butter for variety. Scale up to feed the neighborhood kids.

Makes 1 log

> 1 tablespoon almond, cashew, or sunflower butter or tahini
> 1 celery stick
> 1 teaspoon raisins, currants, or goji berries (optional)
> Your choice of sprouts

Spread the nut butter into the celery stick. Press in the raisins, if using, and top with plentiful sprouts.

GOJI ALMOND BITES

I could snack on salad sprouts by the bushel, but if you are just getting your sprouting game going, almonds and sunflower seeds (make sure you use the seeds, not the green shoots) might just be the thing. These bites will satisfy a sweet tooth and give you a clean boost at a fraction of the cost of store-bought energy bars. Consider making a double batch to keep handy in the freezer. If you don't have sprouted sunflower seeds available, you can swap raw, un-sprouted sunflower seeds or omit them.

Makes about 18 bites

1 cup sprouted almonds
1 cup dried, pitted Medjool dates
½ cup unsweetened shredded coconut
1 tablespoon virgin coconut oil
½ teaspoon lemon zest
½ teaspoon vanilla powder
¼ teaspoon sea salt
¼ cup sprouted sunflower seeds
¼ cup dried goji berries
2 tablespoons raw cacao nibs

1. If the almonds are damp from sprouting, pat them dry with paper towels.
2. In a food processor, combine the almonds, dates, coconut, coconut oil, lemon zest, vanilla, and salt and process until well combined and until the dates are mostly smooth, punctuated by visible bits of nuts. Add the sprouted sunflower

seeds, goji berries, and cacao nibs and pulse to combine but not to break them down. Transfer to a bowl and form the mixture into about 18 (1-inch) balls. Place into a freezer container or zip-top freezer bag and store in the freezer for up to 2 months. Thaw just before eating.

RAW CACAO BROWNIE BITES

Sprouted almonds and a double hit of cacao make these little bites of brownie bliss extra-moist, almost like fudge. Once you have the almonds sprouted, they take under 10 minutes to put together. It will be infinitely worth the investment!

Makes about 12 bites

> 6 tablespoons raw cacao powder
> 1 cup sprouted almonds
> 1 cup dried, pitted Medjool dates
> 1 tablespoon virgin coconut oil
> ½ teaspoon vanilla powder or extract
> ⅛ teaspoon sea salt
> 1 tablespoon raw cacao nibs
> ¼ cup unsweetened dried coconut, cacao nibs, or pink
>   peppercorns, for rolling

1. If the almonds are damp from sprouting, pat them dry with paper towels.
2. Place the cacao powder in a food processor. Add the almonds, dates, coconut oil, vanilla, and salt. Process until the mixture is mostly smooth but with visible pieces of nuts showing. Make sure not to overprocess so you arrive at that sweet spot between brownie and fudge. Add the cacao nibs and pulse just to combine.
3. Transfer to a bowl and form the mixture into about 12 (1½-inch) balls. Put the bites on a large plate and shower with the

dried coconut. Roll the balls in the coconut and pat them to make sure it sticks. Place into a freezer container or zip-top freezer bag and store in the freezer for up to 2 months. Thaw just before eating.

CARDAMOM ROSEWATER HALVAH

These are the flavors of the Middle East, in raw, sprouted form and without the refined sugar that typically defines this sweet treat. You'll need to let the food processor go for up to 5 minutes to get a smooth consistency, so be patient, and if the machine or ingredients start to get hot, take a break and let them cool down for a few minutes.

Makes about 12 balls

1½ cups (about 5 ounces) sprouted sesame seeds
1 cup dried, pitted Medjool dates
½ cup almond flour
2 tablespoons virgin coconut oil
2 tablespoons rosewater
½ teaspoon ground cardamom
⅛ teaspoon sea salt
⅓ cup finely chopped raw pistachios or shredded coconut

1. In a food processor (a mini food processor works well), combine the sprouted sesame seeds, dates, almond flour, oil, rosewater, cardamom, and salt and process until very smooth, about 5 minutes, stopping to scrape the sides several times.
2. Transfer to a bowl and form the mixture into about 12 (1½-inch) balls. It will be sticky, so you may need to wet your hands as you go. Spread the pistachios on a

plate and roll the balls in the pistachios to coat, pressing lightly so they stick. Place into a freezer container or zip-top freezer bag and store in the freezer for up to 2 months. Thaw just before eating.

ACKNOWLEDGMENTS

I would like to acknowledge Denise Mari for turning me on to the plant-based lifestyle in April 1999. Back then, I didn't know what organic was and I thought a vegetarian was someone from California. You inspired me and provided me with knowledge and opportunities to radically improve my life and to create socially responsible businesses. To Oliver Mari, my godson, who has an indomitable will to create.

To my incredible collaborator, Leda Scheintaub, for her brilliance in creating recipes with sprouts that are both delicious and incredibly healthy. Not to mention the late nights, early mornings, and infinite patience in outlining, organizing, and editing my passions.

To my literary agents at Park Fine: Sarah Passick, Celeste Fine, and Anna Petkovich, who helped map out a path of success for this concept.

To my editor at St. Martin's Press, Elizabeth Beier, for hearing my story, immediately eating my sprouts, and committing to sharing the sprout vision with the world. To Hannah Phillips for being there for us and for the loving nudges. Many thanks also to Olga Grlic, Jeremy Haiting, Lisa Davis, Brant Janeway,

Erica Martirano, Kelly Klein, Sara Ensey, Steven Seighman, Naureen Nashid, and Rowen Davis.

To our talented photographer, Clare Barboza, who makes sprouts look gourmet and craveable. And to Jenn LaVardera for keeping our facts straight.

To the incredible teachers and mentors who agreed to be interviewed for the book: Josh Axe, M.D.; Brian Clement, M.D.; Stephen Fiskell; Joel Fuhrman, M.D.; Alan Goldhamer, M.D.; Michael Greger, M.D.; Mark Hyman, M.D.; Joel Kahn, M.D.; Stacy Kennedy; Joseph Mercola, M.D.; Dean Ornish, M.D.; Mehmet Oz, M.D.; and Katie Wells.

To Paulette Cole for inspiring me through everything that she has created at ABC Carpet and Home, my favorite restaurant, abcV, and all the love she shares with the world.

To my teachers and friends in the consciousness and plant-based world: Sahara Rose, David Wolfe, Gabriel Cousens, David Jubb, Doug Graham, John McDougal, Neil Barnard, Viktoras Kulvinskas, Julie Piatt ("SriMati"), Rich Roll, Alejandro Junger, Michael Klaper, John Joseph, and Ari and Noah Meyerowitz.

To my friends at OWN, Oprah Winfrey, Gayle King, Adam Glassman, Raeann Herman and Kelsey Farish for sharing so much love and goodness with the world.

To Yves Behar and Fuseproject for being the best design partners one could ask for.

To Giles Lowe, Arne Lang-Ree, and the team at Spanner for their help in designing products for the masses.

To my friends who inspire me and reflect the truth to me always: Jack Hidary, Tia Kansara, Jenna Lee Prince, Ryan Allis, Ashlee Margolis, Steven Jensen, Joel Seiden, Harry Mcilroy, Gidon Wise, Sonia Jones, Casey Neistat, Michael Franti, Mike Posner, Josh

Kushner, Jeff Rosenthal, Elliot Bisnow, Baruch Gorkin, Yaron Sheba, Hannah Heenan, Mikaela Windham-Herman, Dr. Deb, Brian Herman, Brad Palmer, Dhru Purohit, Myka Mcglaughlin, Debra Winter, Maria Marlowe, Jud Traphagen, Alessandro Piol, Alice Frank, Jay Edlin, Tom Scott, Matt Wiggins, Daniel Schmactenberger, Julia Allison, Jesse Itzler, Randy Komisar, David Krane, Matt Rogers, Mike Harden, Stuart Peterson, Rita and Peter Thomas, Rachel Rossitto, Hannah Heenan, Bill Elkus, Amir Banifatemi, Radha Agrawal, Miki Agrawal, Henry Chalfant, George Naddaff, Lori Herbel, Laurin Seiden, Evan Seiden, Malachy Moynihan, Starielle Hope, and Eli Call.

To my whole Camp Mystic family for showing me what's possible in community.

To the many of you who I unconsciously left out, but you know who you are. Please feel free to accept my apologies in advance and remind me. I am far from perfect.

RESOURCES

The Sprout Book
www.thesproutbook.com
The book's own website, with links to everything related to sprouting, including nutritional information, further resources, and ecommerce.

My Blog
www.dougevans.com

Online Seed Catalogs, Sprouting Jars, Trays and Pots, Fertilizers, and Cleaning Agents

Sprout Guru
www.sproutguru.com

Sproutman
www.sproutman.com

Sproutpeople
www.sproutpeople.org

www.sproutero.com

International Specialty Supply / Sproutnet
www.sproutnet.com

My Patriot Supply
www.mypatriotsupply.com

CropKing
www.cropking.com

True Leaf Market
www.trueleafmarket.com

Amazon.com
ebay.com

Wheatgrass auger juicer
Sproutman
www.sproutman.com

Green plastic produce bags
Debbie Meyer
www.debbiemeyer.com

Further Information on Sprouts
Dietary Guidelines for Americans 2015–2020
https://health.gov/dietaryguidelines/2015/guidelines/

GreenMedInfo
www.greenmedinfo.com

Mercola
www.mercola.com

NutritionFacts.org
www.nutritionfacts.org

Health Centers
TrueNorth Health Center
www.healthpromoting.com

Hippocrates Health Institute
www.hippocratesinst.org

BIBLIOGRAPHY

Adzuki Bean Sprouts

Hardy, Erin. "What's So Special About Adzuki Beans?" Osmia Organics. March 1, 2019. https://osmiaorganics.com/blogs/blog/whats-so-special-about-adzuki-beans.

Jaoude, Marc. "Adzuki Bean Sprouts." Markito Fitness & Nutrition. 2019. https://markitonutrition.com/adzuki-bean-sprouts/.

Petre, Alina. "Adzuki Beans: Nutrition, Benefits and How to Cook Them." Healthline. December 13, 2018. https://www.healthline.com/nutrition/adzuki-beans.

Price, Annie. "Adzuki Beans Can Improve Your Heart, Weight & Muscle Mass." Dr. Axe. June 4, 2016. https://draxe.com/adzuki-beans/.

Staughton, John. "8 Interesting Benefits of Adzuki Beans." Organic Facts. April 9, 2019. https://www.organicfacts.net/health-benefits/other/adzuki-beans.html.

Air Quality

Palermo, Elizabeth. "Do Indoor Plants Really Clean the Air?" Live Science. July 29, 2013. https://www.livescience.com/38445-indoor-plants-clean-air.html.

Alfalfa Sprouts

Cousens, Gabriel. "A Healthy Perspective of Sprouts." Sprout People. Accessed July 28, 2019. https://sproutpeople.org/sprouts/nutrition/science/#gabe.

Johns Hopkins Lupus Center. "Things to Avoid." Accessed July 28, 2019. https://www.hopkinslupus.org/lupus-info/lifestyle-additional-information/avoid/.

Self Nutrition Data. "Alfalfa Seeds, Sprouted, Raw Nutrition Facts & Calories." Accessed July 28, 2019. https://nutritiondata.self.com/facts/vegetables-and-vegetable-products/2302/2.

Alzheimer's Disease

Kameyama T., T. Nabeshima, and T. Kozawa. "Step-Down-Type Passive Avoidance- and Escape-Learning Method. Suitability for Experimental Amnesia Models." *Journal of Pharmacological Methods* 16, no. 1 (1986): 39–52. https://www.ncbi.nlm.nih.gov/pubmed/3747545.

Zhang, Rui, Jingzhu Zhang, Lingduo Fang, Xi Li, Yue Zhao, Wanying Shi, and Li An. "Neuroprotective Effects of Sulforaphane on Cholinergic Neurons in Mice with Alzheimer's Disease-Like Lesions." *International Journal of Molecular Science* 15, no. 8 (2014): 14396–14410. doi:10.3390/ijms150814396.

Arugula Sprouts

Cure Joy. "Health Benefits of Arugula: The Mighty Microgreen." December 7, 2017. https://www.curejoy.com/content/health-benefits-of-arugula/.

Autism

Autism Speaks. "Broccoli Sprouts for Autism? What You Need to Know." October 14, 2014. https://www.autismspeaks.org/expert-opinion/broccoli-sprouts-autism-what-you-need-know.

Otto, Alexander. "Sulforaphane for Autism? Maybe." Clinical Neurology News. May 19, 2018. https://www.mdedge.com/clinicalneurologynews/article/166118/pediatrics/sulforaphane-autism-maybe.

Perlmutter, David. "Sulforaphane Improves Autism Symptoms." Accessed July 28, 2019. https://www.drperlmutter.com/chemical-present-broccoli-vegetables-may-improve-autism-symptoms/.

Autoimmune Diseases

Bocco, Diana. "The Difference Between Lupus and RA." Healthline. November 5, 2018. https://www.healthline.com/health/lupus-and-ra.

Myers, Amy. "5 Things You Can Do to Help Reverse Your Autoimmune Disease That Your Doctor Isn't Telling You." *Huffington Post.* Updated March 23, 2017. https://www.huffpost.com/entry/5-things-you-can-do-to-re_n_9515902.

Basil Microgreens

Hochwald, Lambeth. "9 Microgreens Full of Meganutrients." MNN. July 28, 2015. https://www.mnn.com/food/healthy-eating/stories/9-microgreens-full-meganutrients.

Nordqvist, Joseph. "Why Everyone Should Eat Basil." Medical News Today. Updated January 3, 2018. https://www.medicalnewstoday.com/articles/266425.php.

Nutrition and You.com. "Basil Herb Nutrition Facts." Accessed July 28, 2019. https://www.nutrition-and-you.com/basil-herb.html.

Our Herb Garden. "Basil." Accessed July 28, 2019. http://www.ourherbgarden.com/herb-history/basil.html.

Xiao, Zhenlei, Gene E. Lester, Yaguang Luo, and Qin Wang. "Assessment of Vitamin and Carotenoid Concentrations of Emerging Food Products: Edible Microgreens." *Journal of Agricultural and Food Chemistry* 60, no. 31 (2012): 7644–7651. https://doi.org/10.1021/jf300459b.

Ware, Megan. "Health Benefits of Microgreens." Medical News Today. Accessed February 27, 2017. https://www.medicalnewstoday.com/articles/316075.php.

Beta-Carotene

Alpha-Tocopherol Beta Carotene Cancer Prevention Study Group. "The Effect of Vitamin E and Beta Carotene on the Incidence of Lung Cancer and Other Cancers in Male Smokers." *New England Journal of Medicine* 330, no. 15 (1994): 1029–1035. doi:10.1056/NEJM199404143301501.

Good Inside at Touchstone Essentials. "Dangers of Synthetic Beta Carotene." Accessed July 27, 2019. https://thegoodinside.com/the-dangers-of-synthetic-beta-carotene/.

Hautvast, J. G., K. H. van Het Hof, C. E. West, and J. A. Weststrate. "Dietary Factors That Affect the Bioavailability of Carotenoids." *Journal of Nutrition* 130, no. 3 (2000): 503–506. doi:10.1093/jn/130.3.503.

Heal with Food. "Some Microgreens Contain Even More Beta-Carotene Than Carrots." Accessed July 27, 2019. https://www.healwithfood.org/articles/microgreens-beta-carotene-study.php.

Lester, G. E., Q. Wang, and Z. Xiao. "Assessment of Vitamin and Carotenoid Concentrations of Emerging Food Products: Edible Microgreens." *Journal of Agricultural and Food Chemistry* 60, no. 31 (2012): 7644–7651. doi:10.1021/jf300459b.

Olsen, Natalie. "Benefits of Beta Carotene and How to Get It." Healthline. February 7, 2018. https://www.healthline.com/health/beta-carotene-benefits.

"Women with Higher Carotenoid Levels Have Reduced Risk of Breast Cancer." *JNCI: Journal of the National Cancer Institute* 104, no. 24 (2012). https://doi.org/10.1093/jnci/djs627.

Biotech Crops

ISAAA. "Pocket K No. 16: Biotech Crop Highlights in 2017." Updated October 2018. http://www.isaaa.org/resources/publications /pocketk/16/.

Brain Health

Brown, Helen. "30 Evidence-Based Benefits of Brussel Sprouts." Well-Being Secrets. July 1, 2019. https://www.well-beingsecrets .com/brussel-sprouts-health-benefits/.

Houghton, Christine A., Robert G. Fassett, and Jeff S. Coombes. "Sulforaphane and Other Nutrigenomic Nrf2 Activators: Can the Clinician's Expectation Be Matched by the Reality?" *Oxidative Medicine and Cellular Longevity* 2016 (2016): 1–17. http://dx.doi .org/10.1155/2016/7857186.

Ruhoy, Ilene. "'Sprouting' Is the Healthiest (and Least Expensive) Thing You Can Do for Your Brain Health." Mind Body Green. March 8, 2019. https://www.mindbodygreen.com/articles/health -benefits-of-sprouting.

Zhao, X., L. Wen, M. Dong, and X. Lu. "Sulforaphane Activates the Cerebral Vascular Nrf2-ARE Pathway and Suppresses Inflammation to Attenuate Cerebral Vasospasm in Rat with Subarachnoid Hemorrhage." *Brain Research* 15, no. 1653 (2016): 1–7. doi:10.1016/j.brainres.2016.09.035.

Broccoli Sprouts

Cell-Logic. "5 Amazing Health Benefits of Broccoli Sprouts." May 5, 2018. https://www.cell-logic.com.au/5-amazing-health-benefits -broccoli-sprouts/.

Egner, Patricia A., Jian Guo Chen, Adam T. Zarth, Derek Ng, Jinbing Wang, Kevin H. Kensler, Lisa P. Jacobson, et al. "Rapid and Sustainable Detoxication of Airborne Pollutants by Broccoli Sprout Beverage: Results of a Randomized Clinical Trial in China."

Cancer Prevention Research, June 9, 2014. doi:10.1158/1940-6207. CAPR-14-0103.

Fahey, Jed W., Paul Talalay, and Yuesheng Zhang. "Broccoli Sprouts: An Exceptionally Rich Source of Inducers of Enzymes That Protect Against Chemical Carcinogens." *PNAS* 94, no. 19 (1997): 10367–10372. https://doi.org/10.1073/pnas.94.19.10367.

Lynch, Rhoda, Eileen L. Diggins, Susan L. Connors, Andrew W. Zimmerman, Kanwaljit Singh, Hua Liu, Paul Talalay, and Jed W. Fahey. "Sulforaphane from Broccoli Reduces Symptoms of Autism: A Follow-Up Case Series from a Randomized Double-Blind Study." *Global Advances in Health and Medicine* 6 (2017). doi:10.1177/2164957X17735826.

Nestle, Marion. "Broccoli Sprouts as Inducers of Carcinogen-Detoxifying Enzyme Systems: Clinical, Dietary, and Policy Implications." *PNAS* 94, no. 21 (1997): 11149–11151. https://doi.org/10.1073/pnas.94.21.11149.

NutritionFact.Org. "Broccoli Sprouts." Accessed August 2, 2019. https://nutritionfacts.org/topics/broccoli-sprouts/.

Sifferlin, Alexandra. "Broccoli-Sprout Beverage Can Detoxify Pollutants." *Time.* June 17, 2014. https://time.com/2891178/broccoli-sprout-beverage-can-detoxify-pollutants/.

Singh, Kanwaljit, Susan L. Connors, Eric A. Macklin, Kirby D. Smith, Jed W. Fahey, Paul Talalay, and Andrew W. Zimmerman. "Sulforaphane Treatment of Autism Spectrum Disorder (ASD)." *PNAS* 111, no. 43 (2014): 15550–15555. https://doi.org/10.1073/pnas.1416940111.

Stevens, Jan F., and Claudia S. Maier. "Sources, Metabolism, and Biomolecular Interactions Relevant to Human Health and Disease." *Molecular Nutrition & Food Research* 52, no. 1 (2008): 7–25. doi:10.1002/mnfr.200700412.

Cabbage Sprouts

Bruso, Jessica. "Soluble Fiber in Cabbage." *SF Gate*. Updated December 27, 2018. https://healthyeating.sfgate.com/soluble-fiber-cabbage-4643.html.

Huang, Haiqiu, Xiaojing Jiang, Zhenlei Xiao, Lu Yu, Quynhchi Pham, Jianghao Sun, Pei Chen, et al. "Red Cabbage Microgreens Lower Circulating Low-Density Lipoprotein (LDL), Liver Cholesterol, and Inflammatory Cytokines in Mice Fed a High-Fat Diet." *Journal of Agricultural and Food Chemistry* 64, no. 48 (2016): 9161–9171. https://doi.org/10.1021/acs.jafc.6b03805.

Kubala, Jillian. "9 Impressive Health Benefits of Cabbage." Healthline. November 4, 2017. https://www.healthline.com/nutrition/benefits-of-cabbage.

Mercola, Joseph. "The Latest Superfood: Red Cabbage Sprouts." Mercola. December 26, 2016. https://articles.mercola.com/sites/articles/archive/2016/12/26/superfood-red-cabbage-sprouts.aspx.

Staughton, John. "9 Impressive Benefits of Red Cabbage." Organic Facts. Updated June 21, 2019. https://www.organicfacts.net/health-benefits/vegetable/red-cabbage.html.

Cancer

Champ, Colin. "Sprouts and Cancer—Sulfur, Stress, and Fighting Cancer with Food." ColinChamp.com. February 21, 2017. http://colinchamp.com/sprouts-and-cancer-sulfur-stress-and-fighting-cancer-with-food/.

Edwards, Rebekah. "Broccoli Sprouts: One of Nature's Top Cancer-Fighting Foods." Dr. Axe. January 16, 2018. https://draxe.com/broccoli-sprouts/.

Jockers, David. "6 Ways Broccoli Sprouts Fight Cancer." DrJockers.com. Accessed August 6, 2019. https://drjockers.com/6-ways-broccoli-sprouts-fight-cancer/.

Memorial Sloan Kettering Cancer Center. "Broccoli Sprouts." Updated June 5, 2018. https://www.mskcc.org/cancer-care/integrative-medicine/herbs/broccoli-sprouts.

National Cancer Institute. "Cruciferous Vegetables and Cancer Prevention." Accessed June 7, 2012. https://www.cancer.gov/about-cancer/causes-prevention/risk/diet/cruciferous-vegetables-fact-sheet.

Sun Garden. "Sprouts and Cancer." Accessed August 6, 2019. https://sproutnet.com/sprouts-and-cancer/.

Cardiovascular Health

Cleveland Clinic. "Vegetarianism & Heart Health." Accessed January 11, 2019. https://my.clevelandclinic.org/health/articles/17593-vegetarianism<-><->heart-health.

Harvard Health Publishing. "The Right Plant-Based Diet for You." January 2018. https://www.health.harvard.edu/staying-healthy/the-right-plant-based-diet-for-you.

HealthDay. "Cardiovascular Health Information." Accessed August 9, 2019. https://consumer.healthday.com/cardiovascular-and-health-information-20/.

Kraft, Amy. "10 Superfoods for Heart Health." *Everyday Health*. Updated November 16, 2016. https://www.everydayhealth.com/high-cholesterol/living-with/superfoods-for-heart-health/#choose-superfoods-to-keep-your-heart-healthy.

Marcene, Brandi. "12 Amazing Health Benefits of Bean Sprouts." Natural Food Series. March 25, 2019. https://www.naturalfoodseries.com/12-benefits-bean-sprouts/.

Staughton, John. "10 Best Benefits of Sprouts." Organic Facts. Updated August 8, 2019. https://www.organicfacts.net/health-benefits/seed-and-nut/sprouts.html.

Wicks, Lauren. "New Study Suggests Vegan Diets Are the Most Effective Prevention Against Heart Disease." *Cooking Light*. De-

cember 18, 2018. https://www.cookinglight.com/news/vegan-diet
-heart-disease-prevention-AHA-study.

Celery Microgreens

Aggie Horticulture. "Celery First Used as a Medicine." Accessed August 9, 2019. https://aggie-horticulture.tamu.edu/archives/parsons
/publications/vegetabletravelers/celery.html.

Health with Food. "Celery Microgreens: How to Grow Edible Celery
Seedlings." Accessed August 9, 2019. https://www.healwithfood
.org/grow-indoors/edible-celery-microgreens.php#ixzz5fO19utPx.

Spark People. "Banana vs. Celery." Accessed August 9, 2019. https://
www.sparkpeople.com/food_vs_food.asp?food=26_49_banana
_versus_celery.

Specialty Produce. "Micro Celery." Accessed August 9, 2019. https://
www.specialtyproduce.com/produce/Micro_Celery_2179.php.

Chia Sprouts

Ancient Grains. "Chia Seed History and Origin." Accessed August 9,
2019. http://www.ancientgrains.com/chia-seed-history-and-origin/.

Link, Rachael. "Chia Seeds Benefits: The Omega-3, Protein-Packed
Superfood." Dr. Axe. January 24, 2019. https://draxe.com/chia
-seeds-benefits-side-effects/.

Lonergan, Christy. "Why Everyone Should Try Sprouting Chia Seeds."
Mind Body Green. January 26, 2014. https://www.mindbodygreen
.com/0-12404/why-everyone-should-try-sprouting-chia-seeds
.html.

Neville, Kerry. "Chia Seeds: Tiny Seeds with a Rich History." *Food
& Nutrition*. December 28, 2013. https://foodandnutrition.org
/january-february-2014/chia-seeds-tiny-seeds-rich-history/.

Chickpea Sprouts

University of Arizona College of Agriculture & Life Sciences. "Garbanzo Beans." Accessed August 10, 2019. https://cals.arizona.edu /fps/sites/cals.arizona.edu.fps/files/cotw/Garbanzo_Beans.pdf.

Clover Sprouts

Budryn, G., I. Gałązka-Czarnecka, E. Brzozowska, J. Grzelczyk, R. Mostowski, D. Żyżelewicz, J. P. Cerón-Carrasco, and H. Pérez-Sánchez. "Evaluation of Estrogenic Activity of Red Clover (Trifolium pratense L.) Sprouts Cultivated Under Different Conditions by Content of Isoflavones, Calorimetric Study and Molecular Modelling." *Food Chemistry* 245 (2018): 324–336. https://doi.org /10.1016/j.foodchem.2017.10.100.

Chandler, Brynne. "What Are the Health Benefits of Alfalfa Sprouts?" *SF Gate.* December 2018. https://healthyeating.sfgate.com/health -benefits-alfalfa-sprouts-4406.html.

Corleone, Jill. "Health Benefits of Clover Sprouts." Live Strong. Accessed August 9, 2019. https://www.livestrong.com/article/481381 -health-benefits-of-clover-sprouts/.

International Sprout Growers Association. "Clover Sprouts: A Natural Cancer Fighter." Accessed August 9, 2019. http://www.isga -sprouts.org/2013/01/638/.

Memorial Sloan Kettering Cancer Center. "Red Clover." Updated October 31, 2018. https://www.mskcc.org/cancer-care/integrative -medicine/herbs/red-clover.

Constipation

Yanaka, Akinori. "Daily Intake of Broccoli Sprouts Normalizes Bowel Habits in Human Healthy Subjects." *Journal of Clinical Biochemistry and Nutrition* 62, no. 1 (2018): 75–82. doi:10.3164/ jcbn.17-42.

Dietary Guidelines

National Academies of Sciences, Engineering and Medicine. "Dietary Reference Intakes: Macronutrients." Accessed August 9, 2019. http://nationalacademies.org/hmd/~/media/Files/Activity%20 Files/Nutrition/DRI-Tables/8_Macronutrient%20Summary .pdf.

Office of Disease Prevention and Health Promotion. "2015–2020 Dietary Guidelines for Americans." December 2015. https://health .gov/dietaryguidelines/2015/guidelines/.

Diets

Eberstein, Jacqueline A. "The Atkins Lifestyle." Controlled Carbohydrate Nutrition. Accessed July 27, 2019. http://www.controlcarb .com/ccn-lifestyle.htm.

Weight Watchers. "All About Beans and Lentils." Accessed July 27, 2019. https://www.weightwatchers.com/ca/en/article/all-about-beans -and-lentils.

Disease Prevention

Bernstein, Lenny. "Watercress Tops List of 'Powerhouse Fruits and Vegetables.' Who Knew?" *Washington Post.* June 5, 2014. https:// www.washingtonpost.com/news/to-your-health/wp/2014/06/05 /finally-a-list-of-powerhouse-fruits-and-vegetables-ranked-by-how -much-nutrition-they-contain/?.

Di Noia, Jennifer. "Defining Powerhouse Fruits and Vegetables: A Nutrient Density Approach." *Preventing Chronic Disease* 11 (2014): 1–5. http://dx.doi.org/10.5888/pcd11.130390.

Fenugreek Sprouts

Goenka, Shruti. "14 Amazing Benefits of Fenugreek Sprouts for Skin, Hair and Health." Style Craze. May 16, 2019. https://www

.stylecraze.com/articles/benefits-of-fenugreek-sprouts-for-skin
-hair-and-health.

Goldman, Rena, and Tim Jewell. "Diabetes: Can Fenugreek Lower
My Blood Sugar?" Healthline. Accessed February 27, 2017.
https://www.healthline.com/health/type-2-diabetes/fenugreek
-blood-sugar.

Khan, Kiroz, Kapil Negi, and Tinku Kumar. "Effect of Sprouted
Fenugreek Seeds on Various Diseases: A Review." *Journal of Diabetes, Metabolic Disorders & Control* 5, no. 4 (2018): 119–125.
doi:10.15406/jdmdc.2018.05.00149.

Renee, Janet. "Fenugreek Sprout Nutrition." Live Strong. Accessed August 9, 2019. https://www.livestrong.com/article/226793-fenugreek
-sprout-nutrition/.

Fiber

O'Brien, Sharon. "Top 20 Foods High in Soluble Fiber." Healthline.
June 15, 2018. https://www.healthline.com/nutrition/foods-high
-in-soluble-fiber.

Petre, Alina. "Raw Sprouts: Benefits and Potential Risks." Healthline. February 23, 2018. https://www.healthline.com/nutrition/raw
-sprouts.

Staughton, John. "10 Best Benefits of Sprouts." Organic Facts. July 24,
2019. https://www.organicfacts.net/health-benefits/seed-and-nut
/sprouts.html.

Flax Sprouts

Ibrügger, S., M. Kristensen, M. S. Mikkelsen, and A. Astrup. "Flaxseed Dietary Fiber Supplements for Suppression of Appetite and
Food Intake." *Appetite* 58, no. 2 (2012): 490–495. doi:10.1016/j
.appet.2011.12.024.

Tan, Verena. "Top 10 Health Benefits of Flax Seeds." Healthline.

April 26, 2017. https://www.healthline.com/nutrition/benefits-of
-flaxseeds.

Taylor, Deila. "Sprouted Flax Seeds." Live Strong. Accessed August 9,
2019. https://www.livestrong.com/article/493597-sprouted-flax-seeds/.

Folate

Link, Rachael. "15 Healthy Foods That Are High in Folate (Folic
Acid)." Healthline. May 22, 2018. https://www.healthline.com
/nutrition/foods-high-in-folate-folic-acid.

National Institutes of Health. "Folate: Fact Sheet for Health Professionals." July 19, 2019. https://ods.od.nih.gov/factsheets/Folate
-HealthProfessional/.

Rychlik, Michael, and Sieghard T. Adam. "Glucosinolate and Folate
Content in Sprouted Broccoli Seeds." *European Food Research and
Technology* 226, no. 5 (2008): 1057–1064. https://doi.org/10.1007
/s00217-007-0631-y.

Ware, Megan. "Why Is Folate Good for You?" Medical News Today.
June 26, 2018. https://www.medicalnewstoday.com/articles/287677
.php.

Food Safety

Like any fresh produce that is consumed raw or lightly cooked, sprouts that are served on salads, wraps, sandwiches, and in some Asian food may contain bacteria that can cause foodborne illness. But unlike other fresh produce, sprouts are grown from seeds and beans under warm and humid conditions. These conditions are also ideal for the growth of bacteria, including Salmonella, Listeria, and E. coli. If just a few harmful bacteria are present in or on the seed, the bacteria can grow to high levels during sprouting, even if you are growing your own sprouts under sanitary conditions at home.

Children, older adults, pregnant women, and people with

weakened immune systems (such as transplant patients and individuals with HIV/AIDS, cancer, and diabetes) should avoid eating raw or lightly cooked sprouts of any kind (including onion, alfalfa, clover, radish, and mung bean sprouts).

https://www.fda.gov/Food/FoodborneIllnessContaminants/Buy StoreServeSafeFood/ucm114299.htm.

Dewey-Mattia, Daniel, Karunya Manikonda, Aron J. Hall, Matthew E. Wise, and Samuel J. Crowe. "Surveillance for Foodborne Disease Outbreaks—United States, 2009–2015." *MMWR Surveillance Summary* 67, no. SS-10 (2018): 1–11. http://dx.doi.org/10 .15585/mmwr.ss6710a1external icon.

Newgent, Jackie. "Are Sprouts Safe to Eat?" Academy of Nutrition and Dietetics. April 10, 2019. https://www.eatright.org /homefoodsafety/safety-tips/food/are-sprouts-safe-to-eat.

Pregnancy, Birth, & Baby. "Cleaning and Sterilising Baby Bottles." Accessed December 2017. https://www.pregnancybirthbaby.org .au/cleaning-and-sterilising-baby-bottles.

Sprout People. "Sprout Growing Q & A." Accessed August 9, 2019. https://sproutpeople.org/growing-sprouts/help/.

U.S. Department of Health and Human Services. "Food Safety by Type of Food." Accessed April 1, 2019. https://www.foodsafety .gov/keep-food-safe/food-safety-by-type-food.

U.S. Food and Drug Administration. "Compliance with and Recommendations for Implementation of the Standards for the Growing, Harvesting, Packing, and Holding of Produce for Human Consumption for Sprout Operations: Guidance for Industry." January 2017. https://www.fda.gov/regulatory-information/search -fda-guidance-documents/draft-guidance-industry-compliance -and-recommendations-implementation-standards-growing -harvesting.

Grains

Nordqvist, Joseph. "What Are the Health Benefits of Zinc?" Medical News Today. Updated December 5, 2017. https://www.medical newstoday.com/articles/263176.php.

Oldways Whole Grain Council. "Sprouted Whole Grains." Accessed August 9, 2019. https://wholegrainscouncil.org/whole-grains-101 /whats-whole-grain-refined-grain/sprouted-whole-grains.

Penn State Extension. "Sprouting the Truth About Sprouted Grains." Updated January 18, 2018. https://extension.psu.edu/sprouting -the-truth-about-sprouted-grains.

Grasses

Bar-Sela, G., M. Cohen, E. Ben-Arye, and R. Epelbaum. "The Medical Use of Wheatgrass: Review of the Gap Between Basic and Clinical Applications." *Mini Reviews in Medicinal Chemistry* 15, no. 12 (2015): 1002–1010. https://www.ncbi.nlm.nih.gov/pubmed/26156538.

Kahn, Masood Shah, Rabea Parveen, Kshipra Mishra, Rajkumar Tulsawani, and Sayeed Ahmad. "Chromatographic Analysis of Wheatgrass Extracts." *Journal of Pharmacy & BioAllied Sciences* 7, no. 4 (2015): 267–271. doi:10.4103/0975-7406.168023.

Link, Rachael. "7 Evidence-Based Benefits of Wheatgrass." Healthline. February 21, 2018. https://www.healthline.com/nutrition /wheatgrass-benefits.

Green Pea Sprouts

Encyclopedia Britannica Online. s.v. "Pea." Updated July 1, 2019. https://www.britannica.com/plant/pea.

Hemp Sprouts

Brugnatelli, Viola. "10 Reasons for Eating Hemp Sprouts." Nature Going Smart. Updated December 6, 2017. http://naturegoingsmart .com/10-reasons-eating-hemp-sprouts/.

Burns, Jo. "How to Sprout Hemp Seeds." Hunker. Accessed August 9, 2019. https://www.hunker.com/12467634/how-to-sprout-hemp-seeds.

Canadian Hemp Trade Alliance. "Background: History of Hemp." Accessed August 9, 2019. http://www.hemptrade.ca/eguide/background/history-of-hemp.

History

Chaney, Cathryn. "Life Span for Oak Trees." *SF Gate.* Accessed July 27, 2019. https://homeguides.sfgate.com/life-span-oak-trees-80036.html.

International Sprout Growers Association. "Sprout History." Accessed July 28, 2019. http://www.isga-sprouts.org/about-sprouts/sprout-history/.

Iron

Cavuto Boyle, Katie. "Plant Based Sources of Iron." Food Network. Accessed July 27, 2019. https://www.foodnetwork.com/healthyeats/healthy-tips/2013/06/plant-based-sources-of-iron.

Kohn, Jill. "Iron." Academy of Nutrition and Dietetics. December 14, 2017. https://www.eatright.org/food/vitamins-and-supplements/types-of-vitamins-and-nutrients/iron.

Petre, Alina. "21 Vegetarian Foods That Are Loaded with Iron." Healthline. May 4, 2017. https://www.healthline.com/nutrition/iron-rich-plant-foods.

Vegan Society. "Iron." Accessed July 27, 2019. https://www.vegansociety.com/resources/nutrition-and-health/nutrients/iron.

Kale

Frost, Meredith, and Daniel Rovell. "The Economy of Kale: Leafy Green Is Taking Over." ABC News. August 4, 2014. https://

abcnews.go.com/Business/economy-kale-leafy-green-taking/story?id=24840049.

Martin, Andrew. "Boom Times for Farmers in the United States of Kale." Bloomberg. May 9, 2014. https://www.bloomberg.com/news/articles/2014-05-09/farmers-are-growing-a-lot-more-kale-now-a-census-reports.

Legume and Bean Sprouts

Andrews, Ryan. "All About Lectins." Precision Nutrition. Accessed August 9, 2019. https://www.precisionnutrition.com/all-about-lectins.

Torborg, Liza. "Mayo Clinic Q and A: What Are Dietary Lectins and Should You Avoid Eating Them?" Mayo Clinic. September 14, 2018. https://newsnetwork.mayoclinic.org/discussion/mayo-clinic-q-and-a-what-are-dietary-lectins-and-should-you-avoid-eating-them/.

Lentil Sprouts

Chandler, Brynne. "The Nutritional Value of Sprouted Lentils." Live Strong. Accessed August 9, 2019. https://www.livestrong.com/article/506760-the-nutritional-value-of-sprouted-lentils/.

Livingston, Lindsay. "How to Sprout Lentils." Lean Green Bean. June 20, 2013. https://www.theleangreenbean.com/how-to-sprout-lentils/.

NutritionFacts.Org. "Lentils." Accessed August 9, 2019. https://nutritionfacts.org/topics/lentils/.

Self Nutrition Data. "Lentils, Sprouted, Raw." Accessed August 9, 2019. https://nutritiondata.self.com/facts/vegetables-and-vegetable-products/2472/2.

Microgreens

Fresh Origins. "Microgreen Facts." Accessed August 9, 2019. http://www.freshorigins.com/microgreens-facts/.

Link, Rachael. "What Are Microgreens? Top 10 Microgreens & How to Grow Them." Dr. Axe. October 11, 2017. https://draxe.com /microgreens/.

Mung Bean Sprouts

Busch, Sandy. "What Are the Benefits of Mung Bean Sprouts?" *SF Gate.* Updated December 2, 2018. https://healthyeating.sfgate.com /benefits-mung-bean-sprouts-5176.html.

Fuller, D. Q. "Contrasting Patterns in Crop Domestication and Domestication Rates: Recent Archaeobotanical Insights from the Old World." *Annals of Botany* 100, no. 5 (2007): 903–924. doi:10.1093/ aob/mcm048.

Heuzé, V., G. Tran, D. Bastianelli, and F. Lebas. "Mung Bean (Vigna radiata)." *Feedipedia.* Updated July 3, 2015. https://www.feedipedia .org/node/235.

Martinac, Paula. "How Much Protein Is in Sprouted & Cooked Mung Beans?" *SF Gate.* December 2, 2018. https://healthyeating.sfgate .com/much-protein-sprouted-cooked-mung-beans-6082.html.

Oplinger, E. S., L. L. Hardman, A. R. Kaminski, S. M. Combs, and J. D. Doll. "Mungbean." Alternative Field Crops Manual, University of Wisconsin Extension, Cooperative Extension, University of Minnesota: Center for Alternative Plant & Animal Products and the Minnesota Extension Service. Updated November 21, 1997. https://hort.purdue.edu/newcrop/afcm/mungbean.html.

Tremblay, Sylvie. "Health Benefits of Mung Bean Sprouts." Live Strong. Accessed August 9, 2019. https://www.livestrong.com/article /408757-health-benefits-of-mung-bean-sprouts/.

Mustard Sprouts

Akruti. "17 Amazing Benefits of Mustard Seeds for Skin, Hair and Health." Style Craze. May 30, 2019. https://www.stylecraze.com /articles/amazing-benefits-of-mustard-seeds/.

Omega-3 Fatty Acids

Greger, Michael. *How Not to Die.* New York: Flatiron Books, 2015.

Hull, Mark A., and Milene Volpato. "Omega-3 Polyunsaturated Fatty Acids as Adjuvant Therapy of Colorectal Cancer." *Cancer Metastasis Review* 37, no. 2 (2018): 545–555. doi:10.1007/s10555-018-9744-y.

Link, Rachael. "The 7 Best Plant Sources of Omega-3 Fatty Acids." Healthline. July 17, 2017. https://www.healthline.com/nutrition/7-plant-sources-of-omega-3s.

Mischoulon, David. "Omega-3 Fatty Acids for Food Disorders." Harvard Medical School. August 3, 2018. https://www.health.harvard.edu/blog/omega-3-fatty-acids-for-mood-disorders-2018080314414.

Osher, Y., and R. H. Belmaker. "Omega-3 Fatty Acids in Depression: A Review of Three Studies." *CNS Neuroscience & Therapeutics* 15, no. 2 (2009): 128–133. doi:10.1111/j.1755-5949.2008.00061.x.

Wani, A. L., S. A. Bhat, and A. Ara. "Omega-3 Fatty Acids and the Treatment of Depression: A Review of Scientific Evidence." *Integrative Medicine Research* 4, no. 3 (2015): 132–141. doi:10.1016/j.imr.2015.07.003.

Onion Sprouts

Blissva. "Onions Sprouts: Benefits and How to Grow Onions from Seeds." Eating Sprouts. May 7, 2018. http://www.eatingsprouts.com/onion-sprouts-how-grow-onions-from-seeds.

Organic

Bassil, K. L., C. Vakil, M. Sanborn, D. C. Cole, J. S. Kaur, and K. J. Kerr. "Cancer Health Effects of Pesticides: Systematic Review." *Canadian Family Physician* 53, no. 10 (2007): 1704–1711. https://www.ncbi.nlm.nih.gov/pmc/articles/PMC2231435/.

Baum, Hedlund, Aristei, & Goldman. "R. Brent Wisner to Speak

About Monsanto Trial at Harvard Law School." September 28, 2018. https://www.baumhedlundlaw.com/9-18-wisner-harvard-law-school/.

Hartman Group. "Organic & Natural 2018: A Hartman Group National Syndicated Research Report." 2018. https://store.hartman-group.com/content/organic-and-natural-2018-study-overview.pdf.

Pets

Becker, Karen. "If Your Pet Likes to Munch on Grass, Here's a Safer, Nutrient-Filled Alternative." Healthy Pets. September 6, 2015. https://healthypets.mercola.com/sites/healthypets/archive/2015/09/06/pet-sprouts.aspx.

Protein

Devi, Chingakham Basanti, Archana Kushwaha, and Anil Kumar. "Sprouting Characteristics and Associated Changes in Nutritional Composition of Cowpea (Vigna unguiculata)." *Journal of Food Science and Technology* 52, no. 10 (2015): 6821–6827. doi:10.1007/s13197-015-1832-1.

Kubala, Jillian. "Essential Amino Acids: Definition, Benefits and Food Sources." Healthline. June 12, 2018. https://www.healthline.com/nutrition/essential-amino-acids.

Sibian, M. S., D. C. Saxena, and C. S. Riar. "Effect of Germination on Chemical, Functional and Nutritional Characteristics of Wheat, Brown Rice and Triticale: A Comparative Study." *Journal of the Science of Food and Agriculture* 97, no. 13 (October 2017): 4643–4651. doi:10.1002/jsfa.8336.

Villines, Zawn. "Top 15 Sources of Plant-Based Protein." Medical News Today. April 12, 2018. https://www.medicalnewstoday.com/articles/321474.php.

Radish Sprouts

O'Hare, T. J., D. J. Williams, B. Zhang, L. S. Wong, S. Jarrett, S. Pun, W. Jorgensen, and M. Imsic. "Radish Sprouts Versus Broccoli Sprouts: A Comparison of Anti-Cancer Potential Based on Glucosinolate Breakdown Products." *Acta Horticulturae* 841 (2009): 187–192. doi:10.17660/ActaHortic.2009.841.21.

Seed to Sprout

Bareja, Ben G. "Plant Seed, the Reproductive Organ of the Angiosperm." Cropsreview.com. April 23, 2019. https://www.cropsreview.com/plant-seed.html.

Flournoy, Blake. "What Is a Plant Embryo?" Sciencing. July 25, 2018. https://sciencing.com/what-plant-embryo-4601843.html.

Kay, Zee. "The Parts of a Seed for Elementary Children." Sciencing. April 25, 2017. https://sciencing.com/parts-seed-elementary-children-7334174.html.

Ma, Hong. "Seed Development: With or Without Sex?" *Current Biology* 9, no. 17 (1999): R636–R639. https://doi.org/10.1016/S0960-9822(99)80411-4.

Seeds

Fraser, Carly. "6 Fruit Seeds You Can Eat to Improve Your Health and Prevent Cancer." Live Love Fruit. April 8, 2015. https://livelovefruit.com/6-fruit-seeds-you-can-eat/.

Shoots

Berry, Jennifer. "What Are the Benefits of Chlorophyll?" Medical News Today. Accessed July 4, 2018. https://www.medicalnewstoday.com/articles/322361.php.

Daniluk, Julie. "Five Health Reasons to Eat Sunflower Seeds and Sprouts." Chatelaine. Updated November 1, 2012. https://www

.chatelaine.com/health/diet/five-health-reasons-to-eat-sunflower-seeds-and-sprouts/.

Gordiner, Jeff. "Sunflower Shoots Are a Salad's Secret Weapon." *New York Times.* July 17, 2012. https://www.nytimes.com/2012/07/18/dining/sunflower-shoots-are-a-salads-secret-weapon.html.

Hard, Lindsay-Jean. "Don't Confuse Your Shoots and Sprouts—Here's How They're Different." Food52. March 19, 2016. https://food52.com/blog/16211-don-t-confuse-your-shoots-and-sprouts-here-s-how-they-re-different.

Jaoude, Marc. "Sunflower." Markito Fitness & Nutrition. Accessed August 10, 2019. https://markitonutrition.com/sunflower/.

Kitchen Daily. "How to Eat and Cook Pea Shoots." *Huffington Post.* Updated December 7, 2017. https://www.huffpost.com/entry/pea-shoots_n_1451984.

Miles, Carol A., Justin O'Dea, Catherine H. Daniels, and Jacky King. "Pea Shoots." Pacific Northwest Extension. January 2018. http://cru.cahe.wsu.edu/cepublications/pnw567/pnw567.pdf.

Skin Care

Healthy Blog. "Eating Sprouts: Wonderful Benefits for Your Hair, Skin, and Overall Health." Accessed August 10, 2019. https://foodtolive.com/healthy-blog/eating-sprouts-benefits-hair-skin-overall-health/.

Power of Positivity. "12 Amazing Benefits of Eating Sprouts for Your Body, Hair and Skin." Accessed August 10, 2019. https://www.powerofpositivity.com/benefits-of-sprouts-for-body-hair-skin/.

Rana, Sarika. "16 Benefits of Sprouting and the Right Way to Do It." NDTV Food. Updated June 22, 2018. https://food.ndtv.com/food-drinks/6-benefits-of-sprouting-and-the-right-way-to-do-it-1691887.

Tadimalla, Ravi Teja. "Sprouts: 7 Health Benefits + Nutrition Facts."

Style Craze. March 26, 2019. https://www.stylecraze.com/articles /benefits-of-sprouts-for-skin-hair-and-health.

Talalay, Paul., Jed W. Fahey, Zachary R. Healy, Scott L. Wehage, Andrea L. Benedict, Christine Min, and Albena T. Dinkova-Kostova. "Sulforaphane Mobilizes Cellular Defenses That Protect Skin Against Damage by UV Radiation." *PNAS* 104, no. 44 (2007): 17500–17505. https://doi.org/10.1073/pnas.0708710104.

Soybean Sprouts

Henley, Danielle. "Soybean Sprouts Compared to Mung Bean Sprouts." Hunker. Accessed August 10, 2019. https://www.hunker .com/13427417/soybean-sprouts-compared-to-mung-bean -sprouts.

Leondard, Jayne. "Everything You Need to Know About Lecithin." Medical News Today. Accessed September 5, 2017. https://www .medicalnewstoday.com/articles/319260.php.

McEvoy, Kara. "The Nutrition in Soybean Sprouts." Our Everyday Life. Accessed August 10, 2019. https://oureverydaylife.com/321781 -the-nutrition-of-soy-bean-sprouts.html.

Mercola, Joseph. "How to Get the Benefits of Soy Without All the Health Risks." Mercola. Accessed August 10, 2019. https://www .mercola.com/Downloads/bonus/dangers-of-soy/report.aspx.

NC Soybean Producers Association. "History of Soybeans." Accessed August 10, 2019. https://ncsoy.org/media-resources/history -of-soybeans/.

Self Nutrition Data. "Soybeans, Mature Seeds, Sprouted, Raw." Accessed August 10, 2019. https://nutritiondata.self.com/facts/vegetables -and-vegetable-products/2623/2.

Sulforaphane

Angier, Natalie. "Researchers Find a Concentrated Anticancer Substance in Broccoli Sprouts." *New York Times.* September 16, 1997.

https://www.nytimes.com/1997/09/16/us/researchers-find-a
-concentrated-anticancer-substance-in-broccoli-sprouts.html.

Coyle, Daisy. "Sulforaphane: Benefits, Side Effects, and Food Sources."
Healthline. February 26, 2019. https://www.healthline.com/nutrition
/sulforaphane.

Edwards, Rebekah. "Broccoli Sprouts: One of Nature's Top Cancer-
Fighting Foods." Dr. Axe. January 16, 2018. https://draxe.com
/broccoli-sprouts/.

True Broc. "What Is Glucoraphane?" Accessed July 27, 2019. https://
truebroc.com/what-is-glucoraphanin/.

Wolz, Cathy. "New Ways with Asparagus." American Institute for
Cancer Research. May 10, 2011. https://blog.aicr.org/2011/05/10
/new-ways-with-asparagus/.

Supplements

Arnarson, Atli. "Folic Acid vs Folate—What's the Difference?" Healthline. June 3, 2017. https://www.healthline.com/nutrition/folic-acid
-vs-folate.

ConsumerLab.com. "Multivitamin and Multimineral Supplements
Review." June 22, 2019. https://www.consumerlab.com/reviews
/Multivitamin_Multimineral_Supplements/multivitamins/.

Vitamin C

Chandler, Brynne. "The Nutritional Value of Sprouted Lentils."
Livestrong. Accessed July 27, 2019. https://www.livestrong.com
/article/506760-the-nutritional-value-of-sprouted-lentils/.

Food Facts. "What Are Sprouts Good For?" November 8, 2016.
https://foodfacts.mercola.com/sprouts.html.

Raman, Ryan. "7 Impressive Ways Vitamin C Benefits Your Body."
Healthline. April 18, 2018. https://www.healthline.com/nutrition
/vitamin-c-benefits.

Saul, Andrew W. "Sprouting Hinters from an Indoor (and Outdoor) Farmer." DoctorYourself.com. 2004. http://www.doctoryourself .com/sprouting2.html.

Wright, Howard. "Sprout Nutrition and Vitamins." June 2011. http://www.hakwright.co.uk/rants/sprout-nutrition.html.

Vitamin K

Arnarson, Alti. "20 Foods That Are High in Vitamin K." Healthline. September 6, 2017. https://www.healthline.com/nutrition/foods -high-in-vitamin-k.

Empey, Allison, and Carrie Phillipi. "Why Does My Newborn Need a Vitamin K Shot?" OHSU Doernbecher Children's Hospital. June 26, 2012. https://blogs.ohsu.edu/doernbecher/2012/06/26 /why-does-my-newborn-need-a-vitamin-k-shot/.

Haelle, Tara. "More Parents Nixing Anti-Bleeding Shots for Their Newborns." Scientific American. August 19, 2014. https://www .scientificamerican.com/article/more-parents-nixing-anti-bleeding -shots-for-their-newborns/.

National Institutes of Health. "Vitamin K: Fact Sheet for Health Professionals." National Institutes of Health, Offices of Dietary Supplements. September 26, 2018. https://ods.od.nih.gov/factsheets /VitaminK-HealthProfessional/.

Ware, Megan. "Health Benefits and Sources of Vitamin K." Medical News Today. January 22, 2018. https://www.medicalnewstoday .com/articles/219867.php.

Watercress Sprouts

Di Noia, Jennifer. "Defining Powerhouse Fruits and Vegetables: A Nutrient Density Approach." *Preventing Chronic Disease* 11 (2014): 130390. http://dx.doi.org/10.5888/pcd11.130390.

Li, Z., H. W. Lee, X. Liang, D. Liang, Q. Wang, D. Huang, and

C. N. Ong. "Profiling of Phenolic Compounds and Antioxidant Activity of 12 Cruciferous Vegetables." *Molecules* 23, no. 5 (2018): 1139. doi:10.3390/molecules23051139.

Plated. "Know a Superfood: Why Watercress Is Such a Powerhouse Vegetable." Accessed August 10, 2019. https://www.plated.com /morsel/know-superfood-watercress-powerhouse-vegetable/.

INDEX

Cleveland Clinic Center for
Functional Medicine, 78
Clinton, Bill, 8
clover sprouts, 71–72
Avocado Sprout Boat with Clover
Chermoula, 206
Clover Chermoula, 218
guide for, 102
coco coir, 118, 147
coconut, 16–17
colanders, 139
constipation, 40, 44
Cook, Captain, 5–6
Cornell University, 100
cruciferous vegetables, x–xii, 33,
46–47
cucumber:
Avocado Salad Smoothie, 171
Crunchy Chickpea Chaat with
Two Chutneys and Cashew
Cream, 189–90
Ginger Broccoli Sprout Smoothie,
172
House Sprout Salad, 204–5
Minty Green Pea Gazpacho,
179–80
Quinoa Tabbouleh, 202–3
Sprouts and Kraut, 191

daidzein, 90
daikon radish:
Carrot and Daikon Noodles
with Sunflower Shoots and
Pumped-Up Pesto, 213
sprouts, 76
Kim Cheese Dip, 188
depression, 36, 37
detox, broccoli sprout, 67–68
diabetes, 34, 36, 37, 73, 84
digestion, 25–26, 31, 40, 68, 80
constipation, 40, 44
dips and spreads:
Kim Cheese Dip, 188

Mushroom-Lentil Pâté, 186–87
New Classic Hummus, 183–84
DNA, xi, 34, 45
dogs, 50

Eat Dirt (Axe), 53
E. coli, 116
Edible Schoolyard, 51
epigenetics, 34
estrogen, xi–xii, 60, 72

FDA (U.S. Food and Drug
Administration), 38, 116–17
fenugreek sprouts, 49, 72–73
guide for, 102
fertilizer, 118–19
fiber, 40, 44, 49, 52, 79, 81, 82
fish oil, 35
Fiskell, Stephen, 98–99
flax sprouts, 73–74
guide for, 103
sprouting setup for, 132–33
folate, 32, 38–39, 68, 77
folic acid, 32, 38, 94
food deserts, 9, 13–14, 50–51
FoodSafety.gov, 121
Franklin, Benjamin, 90
free radicals, xi, 38, 44, 48
fruits, 15, 16, 24
powerhouse, 29
Fuhrman, Joel, ix–xiv, 30–31, 57

Garam Masala Lentils, Cauliflower
Rice, Orange, and Cashew
Cream, 207–9
garbanzo beans (chickpeas), 82
see also chickpea sprouts
Gazpacho, Minty Green Pea, 179–80
gelatinous sprouts:
arugula, 61–62
guide for, 103
sprouting setup for, 132–33
chia, see chia sprouts

ABOUT THE AUTHOR

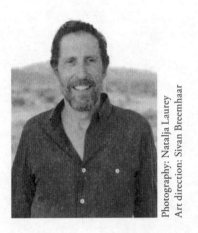

Photography: Natalja Laurey
Art direction: Sivan Breemhaar

Doug Evans is a pioneer in the natural food industry. In 2002 he co-founded Organic Avenue, one of the first exclusively plant-based retail chains in the country. He then created and founded Juicero, the farm-to-glass automatic cold-press juicer, with the mission of bringing fresh-processed foods to the home. Doug lives in the Mojave Desert on a permaculture hot springs oasis.